Conquering   Insomnia

A Comprehensive Guide to Getting a Good Night's Sleep

Dr. Chris F. Miles

Table of Contents

Introduction...........................7

CHAPTER ONE............................ 13
The Science of Sleep
Your Body's Secret Clock.................14
A Sophisticated Ballet...................18
How to Change the Nature of Your
Sleep....................................21

CHAPTER TWO............................31
Potential Causes of Insomnia

CHAPTER THREE..........................37
Developing a sound sleep routine
Developing a pre-sleep routine..........42
Creating a comfortable sleeping
environment.............................45

CHAPTER FOUR.......................... 49
Sleep Hygiene

Night hygiene recommendations...........53
Maintain a regular sleeping routine........54
Within an hour of waking, get some natural light. Wake up quickly! 57
Limit or do without naps..................58
Reduce or stop taking stimulants.......... 60
Don't take certain meds at night........... 61
Do not consume booze three hours or more before going to bed...................62
Don't overeat or be too full before night...63
Regular exercise is important, just not before night................................64
Start a wind-down ritual....................66
In the hour before sleep, ambient lighting should be low................................68
One hour before sleep, turn off all electronics................................... 70
Spend the night in a cozy room.............71
Establish a cozy sleeping atmosphere......73
Avoid being disturbed by your bed companions................................ 75

CHAPTER FIVE................. 79
Promoting healthy sleep through exercise
Promoting sleep through healthy diet......84

CHAPTER SIX.............................87
Insomnia-Prevention and Treatment Recipes
Foot Massage with Lavender.............. 87
Scented pillow for sleep..................90
Sleep-Promoting Sodium Bath...........91
Purple Bath Bomb........................94
Stress Pad................................. 96

CHAPTER SEVEN 99
Retrain Your Brain (Stimulus Control
Therapy)
Treatment for Sensory Control......... 108
Typical Queries (and Answers) and How to
Prepare....................................120

CHAPTER EIGHT.......................125
(Sleep Restriction Treatment) Quality Over
Quantity
Detailed Directions for Sleep Restriction
Therapy....................................131

CHAPTER NINE 143
Mental Health and Sleep
Mindfulness...............................144

Activities for Mindfulness................148
Cognitive Defusion........................152

CHAPTER TEN...........................161
Thinking Differently (Cognitive
Remodeling)
Bad Thoughts.............................165

CONCLUSION............................167

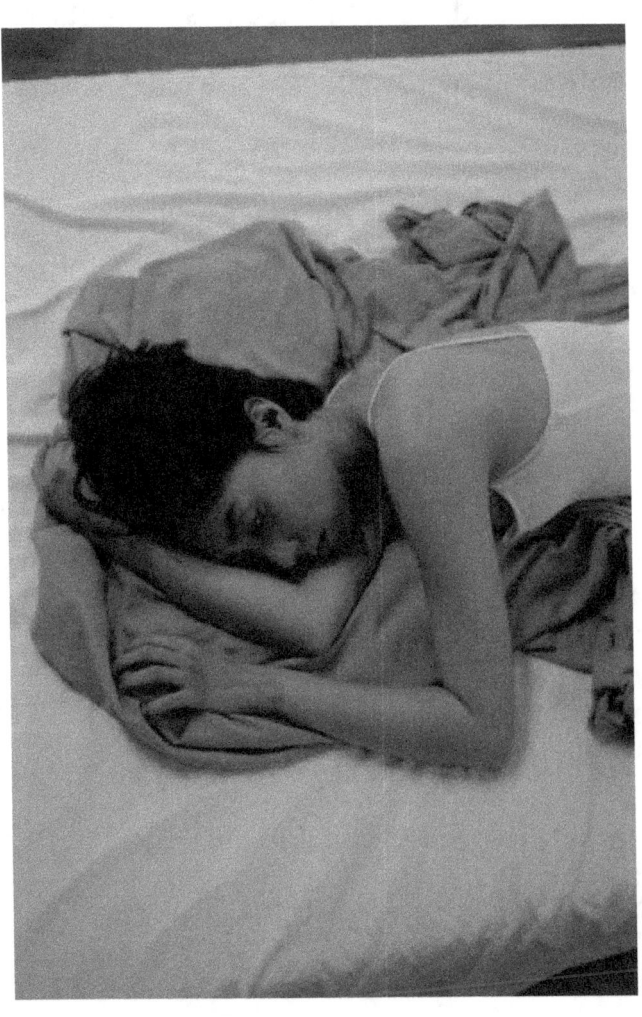

Introduction

It was a dark and sleepless night. No matter how hard she tried, Kaitlyn couldn't seem to get to sleep. She had been struggling with insomnia for weeks now and was beginning to feel desperate for a good night's rest.

Kaitlyn had tried all of the traditional sleep remedies - warm milk, counting sheep, chamomile tea - but nothing seemed to work. She felt drained of all energy, and the lack of sleep was making it difficult to focus during the day. She knew she needed to take action.

So, Kaitlyn decided to take an unconventional approach. She began to explore alternative methods to help her overcome her insomnia.

She researched different relaxation techniques, such as controlled breathing and mindfulness meditation. She also read up on natural sleep aids such as melatonin and valerian root.

Kaitlyn found that the combination of relaxation techniques and natural sleep aids was the key to conquering her insomnia. After a few weeks of consistent practice, she started to notice a difference. She was sleeping for longer stretches of time and falling asleep more rapidly.

Kaitlyn was thrilled with her newfound sleep success. Her energy levels had improved, and she was able to concentrate better during the day.

She was finally getting the rest she needed to live her best life and she was so glad that she had taken the initiative to conquer her insomnia. She was now sleeping soundly every night and felt ready to take on the world.

Life quality is diminished by persistent sleeplessness. People that are sleep deprived are at risk for injuries (including falls and auto accidents), infections, depression, issues with their weight, high blood pressure, heart disease, and diabetes. Ineffective focus and cognitive abilities reduce productivity.

People who are exhausted miss more work and turn down social invitations.The effects on individuals and society are profound.

The goal of treatment is to address the underlying issue that keeps the patient up at night, which may include psychological stress, worry, sadness, heartburn, a persistent cough, menopausal night sweats, frequent urination in older men with enlarged prostates, sleep disturbances, and more.Sleep and its lack have long been a source of worry.

Opium was prescribed for insomnia in ancient Egypt. Opium and its derivatives are obviously dangerous. Hops, lemon balm, skullcap, passionflower, California poppy, and valerian are just a few of the gentler plants that have a long history of use as sedatives.

Hop-filled pillows were purportedly used by King George III and Abraham Lincoln, and this treatment is still advised by herbalists today.

Numerous sedative herbs function on the brain similarly to contemporary sleep aids, according to scientific research, but without the negative side effects. Valerian is the herbal sleep aid with the most study.

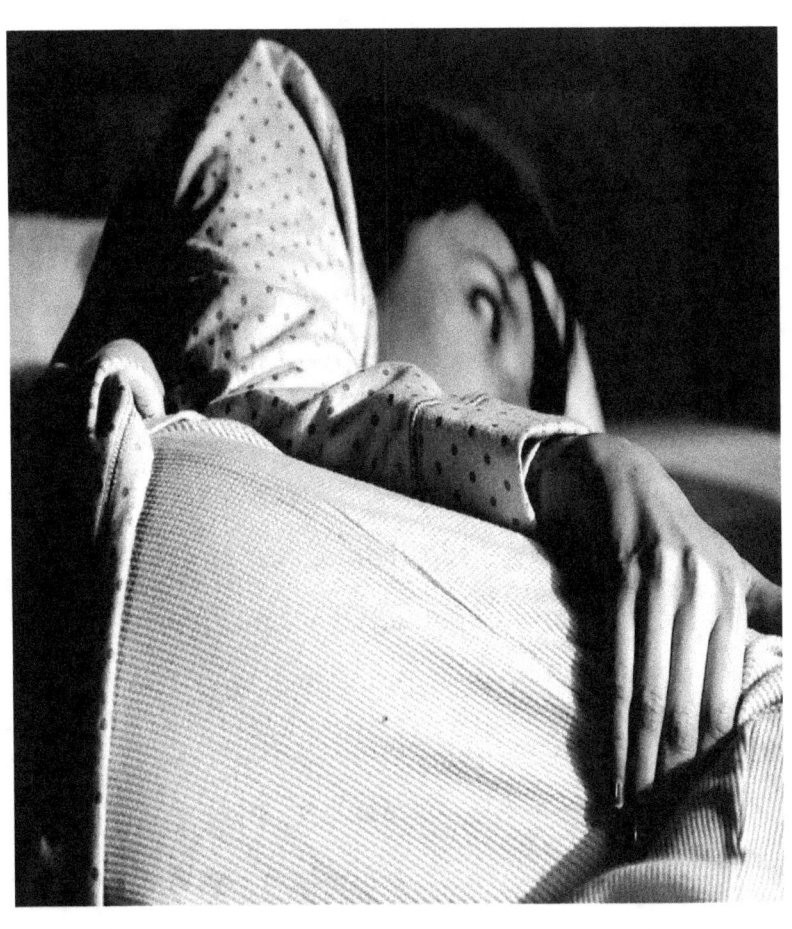

CHAPTER ONE

The Science of Sleep

Being unable to fall asleep, stay asleep, or experience both is a sign of insomnia. It can be caused by many different factors, including stress, medical conditions, unhealthy sleep habits, certain medications, and environmental factors. Insomnia can affect people of all ages and can have a significant impact on quality of life.

In this book, we don't go over every one of these moving components. Rather, we highlight what is most important for this sleep program. Your internal body clock and your sleep drive are the two main actors.

During Sleep, Your body serves as your own particular sleep tracker. Sleep is necessary for life, so your body has an innate drive to get enough sleep in order to survive. It keeps note of how much time you spend sleeping and how much time you spend awake.

Your sleep drive increases when you are conscious; it decreases when you are asleep as the pressure valve opens. Your body will give you signs that it is time to sleep when your desire to sleep is strong.

Your Body's Secret Clock

You can negotiate the cycles of day and night with the aid of your internal body clock. Your circadian rhythm, another name for this biological clock, regulates the timing of your sleep. You can find it inside your cranium. By having an effect on the endocrine system, the nervous system, and the body's internal temperature, your body clock affects your level of wakefulness and sleepiness. The endocrine system is in charge of hormone production.

Melatonin and cortisol are two hormones that are critical for slumber. Your nervous system communicates with your brain to tell it how to react to the surroundings, including when to be alert and when to unwind. Your brain measures changes in your inner body temperature in minuscule fractions of a degree. Your energy and focus are greatly impacted by fluctuations.

When everything is working well, day after day your body clock produces consistent fluctuations in cortisol and melatonin production, nervous system arousal, and core body's temperature. This may manifest itself throughout the day as regular waves of concentration and energy. For instance, you might observe that you have more energy and are more alert and focused in the midday and early evening.

The 24-hour day is marginally shorter than the cycle of the body clock. Actually, the word "circadian" means "about a day" in its precise sense. Remarkably, the human brain is capable of synchronizing these two clocks. The surroundings must help with this.

This was proven by a well-known trial carried out in Europe in the middle of the 1960s. When healthy individuals spent a long time in a basement without windows, their biological clocks began to malfunction. They were no longer in a 24-hour sleep-wake cycle. It appears that exposure to light is a necessary and natural control that keeps us on schedule. When it gets dark, we go to slumber, and when it gets light, we get up. The body clock's capacity to adapt to changes in the environment varies.

Some people easily adapt to external clock changes, such as Daylight Savings Time or travel across time zones. Strong clocks may allow some people to function normally with erratic eating or sleeping schedules.

But others have greater trouble adjusting to changes in the external clock, and may feel a lot more out of kilter when they do not have a regular routine.

A Sophisticated Ballet

Understanding the interaction between the sleep drive and the body clock is important to understanding how sleep works. It is also incredibly beneficial for comprehending your sleeplessness. The internal body clock and the sleep drive are two distinct, independent biological processes, but to support your wake and sleep habits, they must cooperate in a complementary, synchronized way.

We can use the metaphor of meals and appetite to better comprehend this relationship.

Eating three meals a day is customary in many cultures, and these meals are usually eaten in the morning, at noon, and in the evening. Your body desires food at the appointed mealtime when your appetite is balanced. When it's time for food, it will give you signals like hunger pangs. However, your body won't crave eating at the appointed mealtime if your appetite is out of whack—possibly as a result of consuming a large meal or too many snacks. The more consistent you are with your mealtime schedule and the amount of food you eat at mealtime, the more balanced your appetites are. You can tell when it's time to eat without checking the time thanks to this synchronous procedure.

Additionally, it enables you to precisely calculate the amount of food you should prepare so that you won't feel too hungry or filled after eating.

Similar to how mealtime and appetite operate, your body clock and sleep urge do as well. A distinct wake cycle and a distinct sleep cycle are considered normal in our society.

Your body desires sleep at a predictable time when your body clock and sleep drive are in harmony. When it is time for slumber, it will give you cues like sleepiness. Your body will be prepared for sleep during these hours if you maintain a schedule of going to bed at 10 p.m. and waking up at 6 a.m. for a number of months.

This is a synchronous process because you have the resources to sleep when you plan the chance to do so at about the same time every day. Sleeping at your regular time may be difficult if your body clock or sleep drive are thrown off, which could happen if you haven't slept well recently or took a lengthy nap earlier in the day.

How to Change the Nature of Your Sleep

The only thing that affects the sleep drive, as we've already explained, is sleep. As you stay awake longer and longer, your desire to sleep grows stronger and weaker. We've said it already that there are individual variations in how robust our body clocks are, and how sensitive our body clocks are to the environmental cues of light and darkness. Maybe you've convinced yourself that physiological elements of sleep are "hardwired" and unchangeable.

We're happy to inform you! Your actions (what you do) and thoughts (what, when, and where you contemplate) have a significant impact on how your body clock and desire for sleep interact. There are many things you can do to encourage sleep, even though you cannot compel it.

Your biological clock and sleep drive are intended to be supported by actions that encourage restorative sleep. These actions promote changes in sleep patterns that have become dysregulated and support current restorative patterns. They function to improve the body clock, the desire to sleep, and the interaction between the two.

Contrary to behaviors, there is no collection of recommended thoughts that will help you fall asleep. It is not possible to merely will yourself to sleep or to force yourself to think positively about sleep. People who are resting well will tell you they do not think about sleep at all when you check in with them. They appear to have confidence in the sleeping procedure in their overall demeanor. On the other hand, you undoubtedly think about sleep quite a bit, just like the majority of people who have trouble sleeping. Or perhaps your thinking is so active that it keeps you up at night. Either way, these ideas tend to be activating.

Your brain's internal regulators, environmental cues, and your behaviors and ideas interact intricately to produce sleep. These are ever-changing, dynamic interactions that have natural fluctuations. For instance, as you age, your internal body clock adjusts, with adolescence and late adulthood showing the most noticeable differences. In the summer, you receive more sun exposure than in the winter. Events in life will undoubtedly deviate from "ideal" sleep-related behaviors and thought processes. You'll stay up late or get up early to meet deadlines, attend to sick family members, spend time with friends and family, read fantastic novels, or engage in fun video games. We wouldn't want you to avoid reality even if they were!

We urge you to check in with yourself to assess if you are sleeping to live, or living to sleep. Your body is fortunately built to overcome these obstacles. Sometimes you'll go straight back to getting restorative sleep. Your sleep-wake pattern might need to be restored for a few days or weeks at other periods. But rest assured, your body is well equipped to operate in the real world.

Why is there such a widespread problem with bad sleep in our society if we are made to handle these variations? What's going on if your body can't deal with your sleep disruption the way it's supposed to? In the next chapter we will help you comprehend why your brain has not self-corrected, and you are instead stuck in an insomnia spiral.

It is also important to understand the effect insomnia can have on a person's life. People with insomnia may experience fatigue, irritability, difficulty concentrating, and impaired performance at work or school. Insomnia can also lead to depression, anxiety, and an increased risk of accidents.

In order to understand the nature of insomnia, it is important to understand the underlying causes of the disorder. Stress, anxiety, and depression can all be contributing factors. Medical conditions such as chronic pain, breathing problems, and hormone imbalances may also cause insomnia. In some cases, lifestyle factors such as irregular sleep schedules, caffeine use, and smoking can contribute to the problem.

Additionally, certain medications such as stimulants, antidepressants, and allergy medications can cause insomnia. Prolonged daytime sleepiness (your main concern); a red flag that you're not getting enough rest.

Accidents are caused by impaired mental and physical function as well as daydreaming while performing a task (about 5% of Americans fall asleep while driving each month). Impairments in mental and physical function can also lead to clumsiness, slower reaction times, and decreased agility.

Increased risk of work burnout, depression, and anxiety; inability to handle stress; a rise in stress hormones brought on by sleep deprivation; increased pain, including tension headaches; increased inflammation; deteriorating social skills; irritability; reduced alcohol tolerance (plus, sleep deprivation can impair your skills on par with alcohol intoxication); and weight gain (due to hormone changes).

People who aren't getting enough sleep are prone to becoming overly concerned with what's wrong and perceiving peril or vulnerability around every corner. Focusing on promoting and optimizing your healthy sleep instead of fixing or avoiding your urgent sleep issues is one way to learn how to improve your sleep. You'll have more freedom to develop a manageable connection with sleep and a willingness to trust the process if you focus on the elements of healthy sleep. People frequently experience a better feeling that results in increased confidence and success (and, yes, even enjoyment) with sleep when they change their focus in this way.

Keep in mind that knowing what you want (healthy slumber) will help you get it!

In order to understand the nature of insomnia, it is important to understand the underlying causes of the disorder. Stress, anxiety, and depression can all be contributing factors. Medical conditions such as chronic pain, breathing problems, and hormone imbalances may also cause insomnia. In some cases, lifestyle factors such as irregular sleep schedules, caffeine use, and smoking can contribute to the problem. Additionally, certain medications such as stimulants, antidepressants, and allergy medications can cause insomnia.

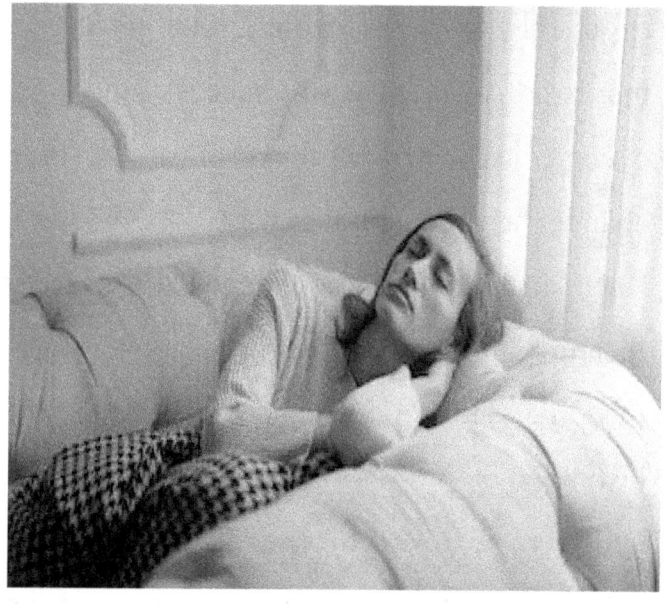

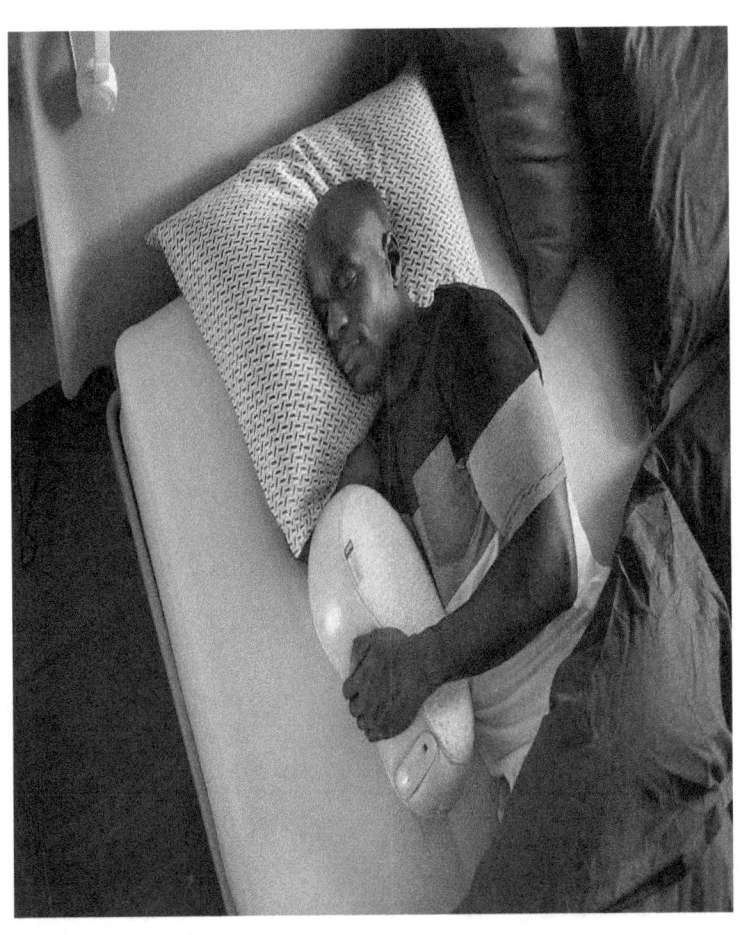

CHAPTER TWO

Potential Causes of Insomnia

1. Stress and Anxiety: Stress and anxiety two of the most common causes of insomnia. Stress can be caused by a variety of things, such as work, family, or financial concerns. Anxiety can be caused by worrying about the future or ruminating on the past. When people are dealing with high levels of stress or anxiety, their bodies become aroused, making it difficult for them to relax and fall asleep.

2. Poor Sleep Habits: Creating a regular sleep schedule and sticking to it can help you get the sleep you need. Poor sleep habits, such as staying up late or sleeping in, can interfere with your body's natural sleep-wake cycle and make it harder to fall asleep and stay asleep.

3. Caffeine: Caffeine is a stimulant and can interfere with your body's ability to fall asleep. Caffeine can be found in coffee, tea, energy drinks, and soft drinks. It is important to limit your caffeine intake and avoid consuming it too close to bedtime.

4. Alcohol: Alcohol is often used as a sleep aid, but it can actually interfere with sleep. While alcohol can help you

fall asleep more quickly, it can cause you to wake up during the night and have difficulty falling back asleep.

5. Medical Conditions: Certain medical conditions, such as asthma, depression, and chronic pain, can interfere with your ability to fall asleep and stay asleep. If you are dealing with a medical condition, talk to your doctor about how it may be impacting your sleep.

6. Medications: Some medications, such as those used to treat colds and allergies, as well as certain antidepressants, can cause insomnia. Talk to your doctor if you think a medication may be interfering with your sleep.

7. Hormones: Changes in hormone levels, such as those that occur during pregnancy or menopause, can cause insomnia. Talk to your doctor if you think hormones may be a factor in your insomnia.

8. Environmental Factors: Environmental factors, such as noise, light, and temperature, can make it difficult to fall asleep and stay asleep. Creating a dark, quiet, and cool bedroom environment can help you get the rest you need.

9. Unhealthy Lifestyle: An unhealthy lifestyle, such as not getting enough exercise, eating an unhealthy diet, or smoking, can interfere with your ability to get a good night's sleep. Making

changes to your lifestyle can help improve your sleep.

10. Shift Work: Working night shifts or rotating shifts can disrupt your body's natural sleep-wake cycle, making it difficult to fall asleep and stay asleep. If you work shifts, talk to your doctor about ways to help you get the rest you need.

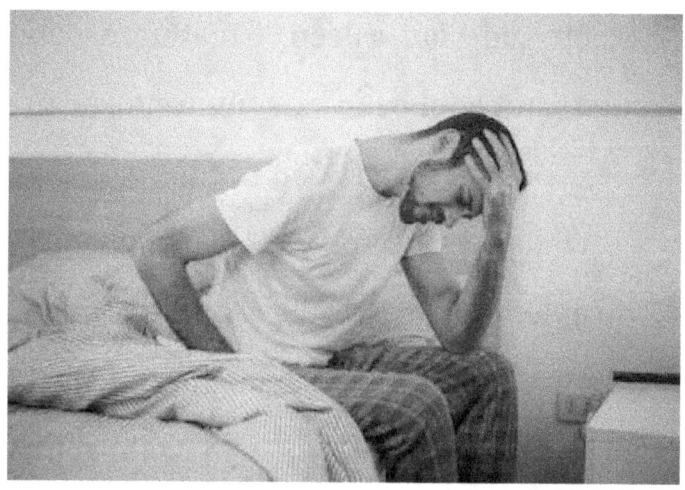

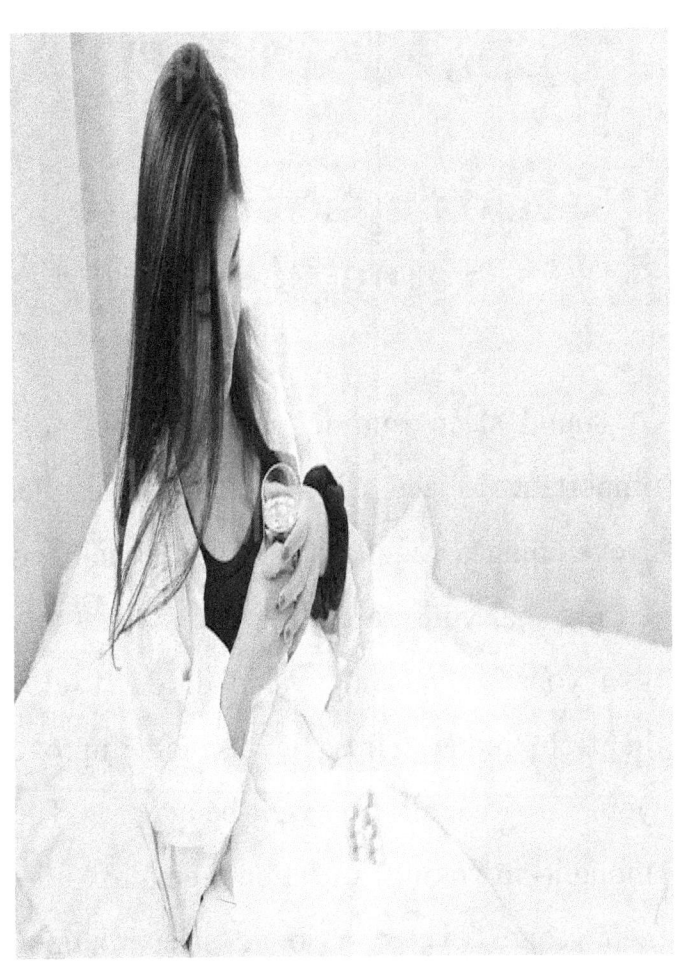

CHAPTER THREE

Developing a sound sleep routine.

A sound sleep routine is one of the most important aspects of a healthy lifestyle. Developing a regular sleep routine helps to ensure that you are getting enough rest and that your body is in top condition. It also helps to reduce stress levels and improve your overall well-being. The thought-provoking question remains how can I one develop a sound sleep routine? The following ideas may be of help.

Establish a sleep schedule

Establishing a consistent sleep schedule is one of the most important habits for good sleep. Going to bed and waking up around the same time each day helps to regulate your body clock and can help you fall asleep more quickly.

Avoid caffeine and nicotine

Caffeine and nicotine are stimulants and can interfere with sleep. Avoid these substances at least 6 hours before bedtime.

Avoid long naps during the day

Naps can be helpful to some people but taking a nap too close to bedtime can disrupt your sleep schedule. Try to limit your naps to no more than 30 minutes and avoid napping after 3 pm.

Exercise regularly

Regular exercise can help promote better sleep. Try to get at least 30 minutes of exercise per day during the day or early evening.

Avoid large meals and alcohol before bed

Eating a big meal close to bedtime can lead to indigestion and discomfort, making it harder to fall asleep. Alcohol can also interfere with sleep patterns.

Create a relaxing bedtime routine

Creating a relaxing bedtime routine can help to signal to your body that it is time to sleep. This could include taking a warm bath, reading a book, listening to soothing music, or doing some light stretching.

Make your bedroom a sleep-friendly environment

Make sure your bedroom is dark, quiet and cool. Remove any distractions such as electronics and reduce any noise.

Avoid screens before bed

The blue light that is emitted from screens can interfere with your body's natural sleep cycle. Try to avoid screens at least an hour before bed.

Take time to wind down

Try to avoid stressing activities before bed and give yourself some time to wind down and relax.

Talk to your doctor

If you are still having difficulty sleeping, talk to your doctor. They may be able to provide additional advice or treatment options to help you get the rest you need.

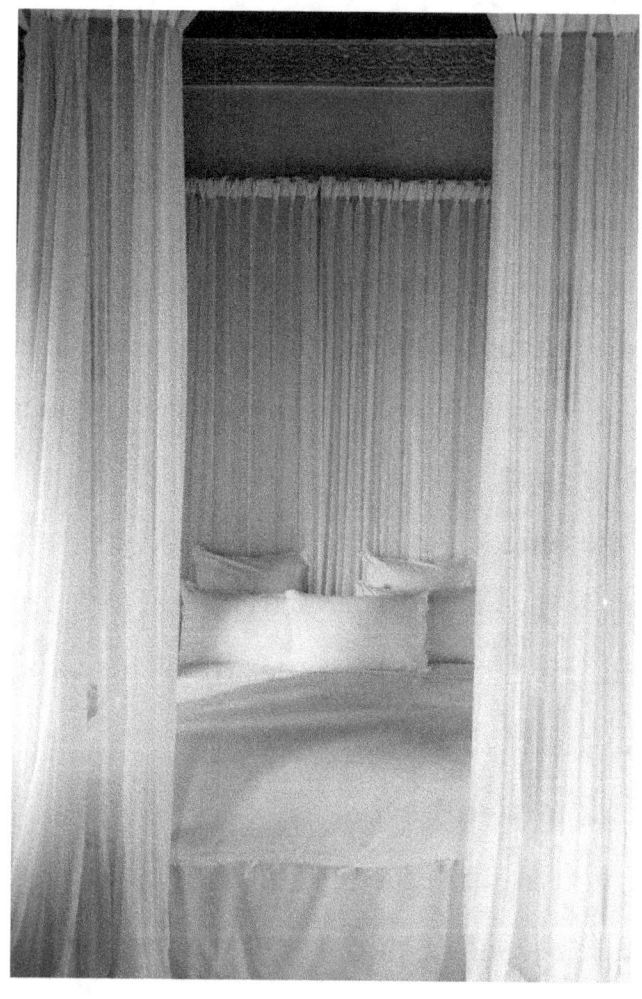

Developing a pre-sleep routine

A pre-sleep routine is an activity or ritual which is performed consistently before bed. The following are some pre-bedtime routine that can get you in some sleep mode.

1. Set aside some time before bed: Set aside at least 30 minutes before bed each night to focus on your pre-sleep routine. This will help you get into a calmer, more relaxed state before bed.

2. Dim the lights: Dim the lights in your bedroom to create a more calming atmosphere. This will help your body recognize that it's time to start winding down.

3. Drink some tea: A cup of herbal tea can be a great way to help you relax before bed. Avoid caffeine for at least four hours before sleep time.

4. Take a warm bath or shower: Taking a warm bath or shower can help your body relax and prepare itself for sleep.

5. Meditate: Take a few minutes to meditate and focus on your breathing. This will help your mind and body relax and ease into sleep mode.

6. Stretch: Doing some gentle stretching can help loosen up your muscles and help you relax.

7. Avoid screens: Avoid watching television or using your phone or laptop for at least an hour before going to bed. The light from screens can interfere with your sleep.

8. Journal: Writing down your thoughts and worries can help clear your mind and help you relax.

9. Read a book: Reading a book is a great way to help you wind down and relax before bed.

10. Get into bed: Once you're ready, get into bed and settle down for the night.

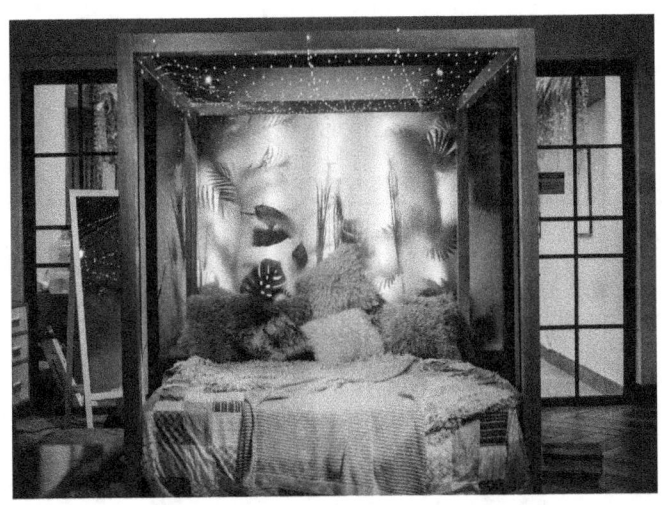

Creating a comfortable sleeping environment

Creating a comfortable and relaxing sleeping environment is key to getting a good night's sleep. To ensure that your sleeping environment is conducive to sleep, there are a few things that you can do.

Keep the room cool

To create a comfortable sleeping environment, keep the room temperature cool. Aim for a temperature of around 65-68 degrees Fahrenheit.

Use comfortable bedding

Invest in comfortable bedding that is made out of breathable fabric. Choose a mattress that is comfortable and supportive.

Choose the right pillow

Select a pillow that is supportive and comfortable. Choose a pillow that fits your sleeping style and that provides enough support for your neck and head.

Use blackout curtains

Block out distracting light and noise by using blackout curtains or shades.

Remove distractions

Remove any electronics or other distractions from your bedroom to help you relax and fall asleep more quickly.

Make sure the room is quiet

Invest in a white noise machine or earplugs to help block out any disruptive noise.

Add soothing scents

Use essential oils, scented candles, or diffusers with calming scents to help create a relaxing atmosphere.

Stick to a routine

Create a consistent bedtime routine that you can stick to each night to help signal to your body that it is time to sleep.

Add comfortable decor

Choose decor that is comfortable and relaxing, such as soft blankets, pillows, and rugs.

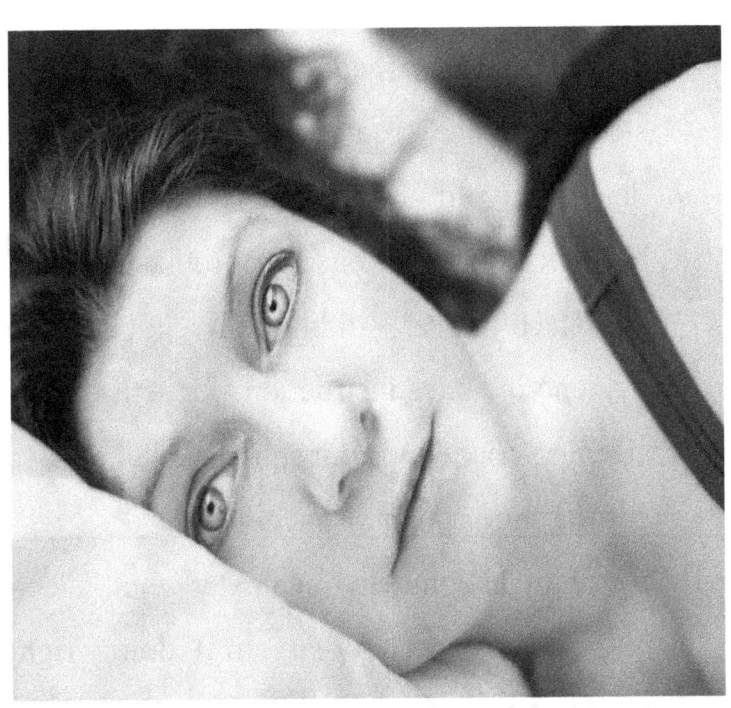

CHAPTER FOUR

Sleep Hygiene

The majority of recommendations for good sleep hygiene center on what you can do—or avoid doing—to influence your biological clock and its synchronization with the sleep drive. Additionally, good sleep hygiene includes instructions for setting up a sleeping-friendly atmosphere, such as a comfortable bed and space.

Some questions to evaluate your sleep hygiene include: "What am I doing right now to support my sleep?" and "What am I doing right now that could disrupt my sleep?" Finding well-intentioned but sleep-interfering behaviors can be made easier by taking into account both viewpoints.

Sleep hygiene is comparable to oral hygiene habits that promote healthy teeth and gums, such as brushing, flossing, and limiting sugary foods. Even if you practice excellent dental hygiene, you can still develop cavities.

When you visit the dentist, you anticipate hearing instructions to keep brushing and flossing, but you do not anticipate hearing that maintaining or enhancing your dental hygiene will eliminate the cavity. The cavity is a different problem that needs extra attention.

The symptoms of chronic sleeplessness and other sleep issues are similar. While you should practice good sleep hygiene, your persistent sleep issues necessitate the inclusion of CBT-I techniques like stimulus control or sleep restriction.

It's interesting to note that individuals with sleep issues frequently struggle with sleep hygiene and are more likely to engage in activities that disturb sleep, like naps or drinking alcohol before bed. Although there is no clear explanation for why this is the case, we have come to believe that people who have trouble sleeping are more reactive to sleep issues. They pay closer attention to any sleep disruptions they experience and feel more pressure to "fix" them. These well-intentioned attempts to address the issue or make up for sleep deprivation frequently run contrary to recommendations for good sleep hygiene and even worsen the situation.

We encourage you to use this chance to change your attention from addressing or avoiding your short-term sleep problems to promoting and optimizing your long-term healthy sleep.

In this chapter, we'll go over the most popular rules for good sleep hygiene and help you determine how ready you are to adjust your habits or your sleeping environment in order to comply with these rules.

Some of these adjustments will entail adding behaviors (like creating a bedtime ritual) while others will entail eliminating behaviors (like quitting drinking before bed). In either case, we are discussing behavioral transformation, which can be difficult. So that you can thrive, we also provide some general advice.

Night hygiene recommendations

Any recommendation can help you change your behavior and keep it changed if you comprehend the reasoning behind it. Due to the fact that all of the behavioral programs in this book, including sleep hygiene, are justified by our knowledge of sleep physiology, we think it is crucial to learn about it.

So, in addition to reviewing each recommendation for good sleep hygiene, we will also discuss its significance. The main takeaway is that if you can get out of your own way, your body will automatically self-regulate, resulting in dependable, restorative sleep.

Maintain a regular sleeping routine

By providing environmental cues like your first exposure to light at the same time every day, a consistent schedule helps your biological clock function properly.

On the other hand, a fluctuating timetable throws off your body clock and makes it work harder to keep regular wake and sleep cycles.

Your body clock depends on a sleep routine not only for this night but also for the following nights and the nights after that as the body clock develops this rhythm over the course of weeks and months.

The most crucial thing is to wake up at the same hour every day. Your body will maintain its rhythm if you rise up at the same time every day, regardless of what time you went to bed the previous night. For instance, if you consistently wake up at 7 a.m., your sleep drive will be at the same location at 11 p.m. every night, increasing the likelihood that you will have a consistent bedtime when life does not get in the way.

No matter how sleepy you feel, even on weekends, we strongly advise that you try to wake up between thirty and forty-five minutes before your goal time. Of course, your wake time will be even less variable when you're participating in a stimulus control or sleep limitation program.

A regular sleep is also beneficial, though there will probably be some variation. We do not want you to become a slave to sleep, so we prefer that you engage in meaningful activities even if this results in variability in your bedtime. For instance, you might have an evening engagement that keeps you up later than usual.

Additionally, we usually advise against going to bed at your target time if you are not tired because this will set you up for lying in bed awake. So, while accepting some variability, we advise you to set a target bedtime and work to keep consistency. Remember that your body will function more smoothly if you get up at your regular hour even after a late night.

Within an hour of waking, get some natural light. Wake up quickly!

Making the transition from sleep to wakefulness as soon as possible is beneficial. This is similar to rapidly removing a Band-Aid from your skin; the quicker you adjust, the quicker you get through any discomfort.

This entails restraining yourself from hitting the sleep button. Additionally, it implies that even if you wake up earlier than expected, it is preferable to get up than to lie in bed and drift off to sleep. Getting some natural light in the first hour after getting up also helps. Light will signal your body schedule to begin your wake cycle for the day; for instance, it will inhibit the production of the hormone melatonin, which serves as a cue for sleepiness.

If bright natural light is not available when you need it, think about using a light source that has a spectrum similar to that of natural sunshine.

Limit or do without naps

Napping can mess with your body clock and reduce your desire to sleep, making it difficult to get to sleep and remain asleep. We've discovered that, for some people, even passing out for a few seconds appears to mess with the body clock. These fleeting moments of sleep appear to tell the brain that it's time to be awake, even when you're not at all rested. If you decide to take a siesta, try to schedule it for no longer than twenty to thirty minutes and no later than midday.

If you frequently fall asleep right before bed, we strongly advise you to find ways to reduce the likelihood of this happening.

For instance, you might decide to sit upright in a chair rather than recline on a plush couch in the early evening, or you might decide to briskly walk to the water fountain if your eyelids start to get heavy while you're sitting at your desk.

Reduce or stop taking stimulants

Any drug that stimulates your nervous system is a stimulant. Caffeine, sugar, and nicotine are a few examples of usual stimulants. If ingesting these, it is best to do so early in the day, before midday. Be aware of sources of caffeine that are less apparent, such as medications (such as Excedrin, Midol, or decongestants) and smoothies with "energy boosts," in addition to the obvious sources, such as coffee, tea, soda, and energy drinks. Stimulants should be avoided or used less frequently to enable your body clock to function normally. By prolonging the time that your nervous system is active, stimulant use affects your body clock and may cause it to become out of phase with your sleep drive (refer back to figure 2.1 for a better grasp of this).

Don't take certain meds at night

Caffeine-containing medications have already been discussed, but even those without caffeine can alter your wakefulness and sleepiness. The most frequent over-the-counter offenders may be decongestants because of their stimulating nature.

Additionally, we have dealt with patients who took stimulant antidepressants like Wellbutrin or stimulants like Adderall or Ritalin too late in the day. A drug that causes sleepiness in one person may cause alertness in another, and vice versa.

To find out if you can shift potentially stimulating medications to earlier in the day and more sedating medications to later in the day, check the common side effects of your medications and speak with your doctor.

Do not consume booze three hours or more before going to bed

Alcohol may aid in falling asleep, but because your body is focused on processing the alcohol rather than resting and recharging your body and brain, it disrupts the structure of slumber. Additionally, since alcohol is a muscular relaxant, it may make your airway more likely to soften, which is worrisome if you have sleep apnea.

Don't overeat or be too full before night.

Aim to have a balanced appetite before night. A snack before night can be beneficial. Although high carbohydrate/low protein snacks are frequently advised, some of our clients discover that the opposite—highprotein/low carbohydrate—helps them sleep through the night.

Avoid overeating before bed, whether you snack or eat a late meal.

Your body needs to have enough food in your small intestine to allow it to relax into sleep without having to work hard to digest it.

In addition, lying down immediately after eating can cause acid reflux or aggravate it, and acid reflux can disrupt your sleep even if you are totally unaware of its presence.

Regular exercise is important, just not before night.

Regular physical activity serves as a strong slumber anchor. Excess stress hormones like cortisol and adrenaline, which can prevent your body clock from establishing and maintaining slumber, can be eliminated through exercise. Exercise also causes your body temperature to increase internally, and timing your workout to coincide with your body's natural rise in temperature can help your body clock even more. Exercise four to five hours before bedtime for the best help with sleep. If you work out at a different time of the day, think about doing some light exercise (like jumping jacks or climbing steps) four to five hours prior to bed to create this core heat.

It is advised that you avoid exercising right before nighttime to prevent a temperature spike that might disrupt your sleep.

Start a wind-down ritual

It is crucial that you set aside time to support the transition from wake to sleep, as opposed to our recommendation that you rapidly transition from sleep with a quick wakeup.

People who demand too much of their brains are frequently encountered; they believe they should be able to work nonstop all day and night and then fall asleep at a moment's notice.

Our minds require a more gradual calming down. A wind-down routine that lasts twenty to sixty minutes will support your body clock in cueing your body to slumber.

We advise you to select calming tasks and perform them in low light. Examples include reading, doing some light stretching, listening to calming music, or taking up a quiet pastime like knitting.

Consider blocking the blue light on your screen if you are unwilling to switch off your screens (phone, tablet, television, or computer) during your wind-down ritual (see below).

There are many individual variations in everything we cover in this book, so we urge you to carefully consider what activities are most likely to help you unwind and prepare for slumber.

Reading a gripping book, doing crossword puzzles, or Sudoku tasks may be just what you need to relax or they may be too stimulating. Writing in a journal can either calm you down or get you fired up as you reflect on your day and leave it behind you.

In the hour before sleep, ambient lighting should be low

Prior to the invention of electricity, most evenings were passed in darkness. Today, we remain indoors for extended periods of time after sunset in environments lit by artificial light, which disrupts our circadian rhythm.

The brain receives the incorrect message from lights, which tells it to remain awake and active. For instance, darkness signals your body to make melatonin, a hormone that induces drowsiness and plays a role in the design of your sleep cycle. Before going to bed, dimming or darkening your surroundings will help with this procedure.

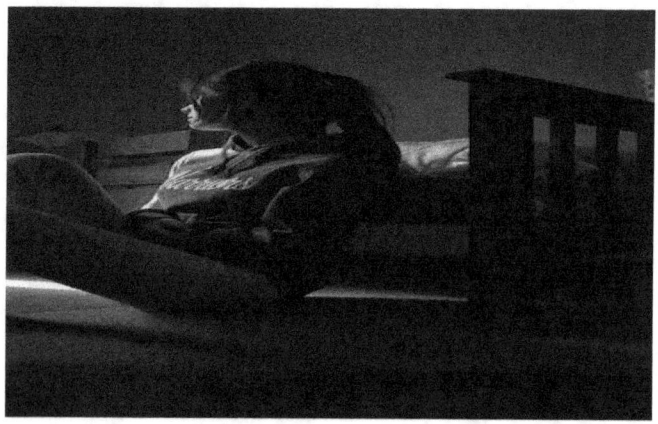

One hour before sleep, turn off all electronics

The enemy of slumber is technology! They generate dazzling light and energizing images, which work against what your body needs to fall asleep and remain asleep. The best course of action is to limit your use of these gadgets to the daylight hours.

Since blue light suppresses melatonin production more than other light wavelengths, you should take steps to block the blue light rays from your device if you're not ready to take a (temporary) break from technology before bed.

You can buy an orange gel to cover your device with or use blue-blocking sunglasses in addition to downloading applications that filter out these particular light wavelengths.

Spend the night in a cozy room

As your body's requirements shift throughout your lifespan, comfort will become a different lens.

Examine your bed in terms of the firmness or softness of the mattress you desire, as well as the degree of warmth or coolness the mattress and your bedding offer.

To find helpful adjustments for your bed or bedding, pay attention to your comfort when you slumber in other beds (like in a hotel or at a friend's or family member's house).

If buying a new mattress is not feasible, you might be able to add a less expensive "topper" to your existing mattress to get the desired sleeping surface.

We don't intend to imply that you require the "perfect" mattress; keep in mind that our goal is to promote adaptability and the capacity to sleep in a variety of settings.

However, we have worked with a few individuals who were attempting to sleep in a chair or on a sofa, and it was evident that this level of discomfort was interfering with their ability to fall asleep.

Establish a cozy sleeping atmosphere

The majority of people will find that a dark, peaceful, well-ventilated bedroom with a cozy temperature is ideal. However, if you spent a long time in a metropolis, complete quiet might be so foreign to you that white noise might help you sleep better.

Also keep in mind that we advise you to use "white noise," which is reliable. As the broadcast switches between programs or between programming and commercials while you sleep with the TV or radio on, the volume will change frequently throughout the night. Even if you aren't fully awakened, these volume changes can cause you to wake up earlier and cause less restorative sleep.

Consider using earplugs, a noise generator, or an eye mask if your surroundings are too bright or loud. These cheap tools can be very beneficial, but they can also have the opposite effect. We have worked with people whose rituals for creating the perfect sleeping environment were so elaborate that they actually made them more stressed and arousable, especially when things went wrong, like when they forgot their eye mask when traveling.

Avoid being disturbed by your bed companions

A crucial aspect of good sleep hygiene is striking a balance between your requirements and those of your partner, kids, or pets. Consider sleeping alone for a while to see if your sleep improves if your bedmates kick, snore, fidget, jump in and out of bed, or (in the case of animals) slumber on your head.

Then, you can decide for yourself whether the advantages of sharing a bed with your partner (or partners) exceed the drawbacks.

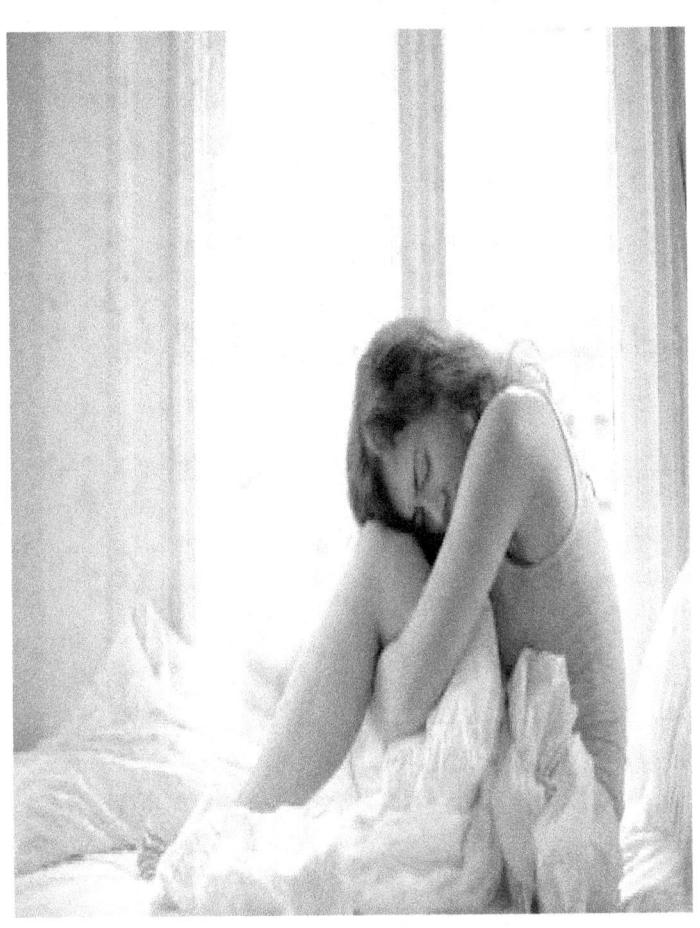

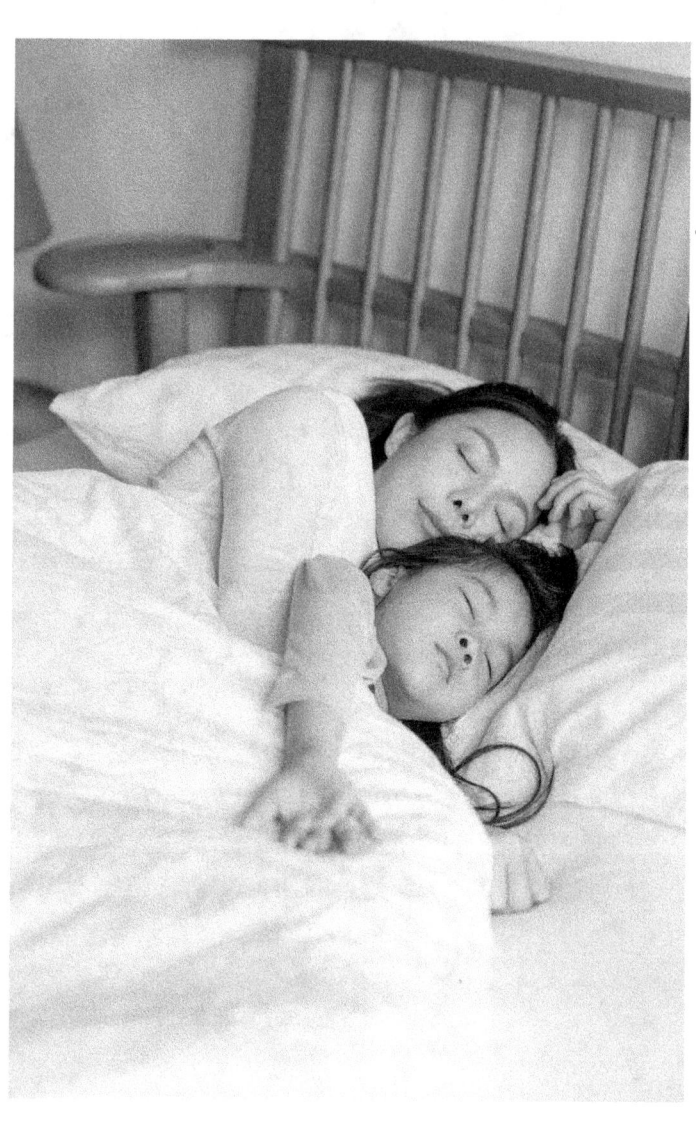

CHAPTER FIVE

Promoting healthy sleep through exercise

Exercise has been proven to be an effective way to improve sleep quality and quantity. Regular exercise helps to regulate the body's circadian rhythm, which is the body's natural cycle of sleep and wakefulness.

By exercising during the day, the body is better able to recognize the difference between day and night, and it can more easily transition between them.

Exercise also helps to reduce stress and anxiety by releasing endorphins into the body. This can help reduce the amount of time it takes to fall asleep and can also improve the quality of sleep.

Exercise can also help to regulate body temperature, which is important for a good night's sleep. When the body is too warm, it can make it difficult to fall asleep. Exercising in the evening can help lower the body's temperature and make it easier to fall asleep.

Exercise can improve the quality of the deep sleep the body needs for rest and restoration. Deep sleep is essential for the body to repair itself and to function properly. Regular exercise can help the body achieve deep sleep more often and more quickly.

In summary, regular exercise can have a positive effect on sleep by helping to regulate the body's circadian rhythm, reducing stress and anxiety, controlling body temperature, and helping the body achieve deep sleep.

Some exercises that promote sleep include;

1. Stretching: Stretching can help to relax the body and release tension which can help improve sleep.

2. Yoga: Yoga has been shown to reduce stress and improve sleep by calming the mind and body.

3. Meditation: Practicing meditation can help clear the mind and reduce stress, allowing for better sleep.

4. Breathing Exercises: Controlled breathing exercises can help reduce stress, relax the body, and improve sleep.

5. Cardio Exercise: Aerobic exercise such as running, swimming, or cycling can help to tire the body, allowing for better sleep.

6. Strength Training: Strength training can help to reduce stress and improve sleep by tiring the body and releasing endorphins.

7. Tai Chi: Tai chi is a slow, gentle form of exercise that can help to reduce stress, relax the body, and improve sleep.

8. Walking: Walking can help to reduce stress, tire the body, and improve the quality of sleep.

9. Swimming: Swimming is a low-impact exercise that can help to relax the body and reduce stress, leading to better sleep.

10. Pilates: Pilates is a low- impact exercise that can help to strengthen the body, release tension, and improve sleep.

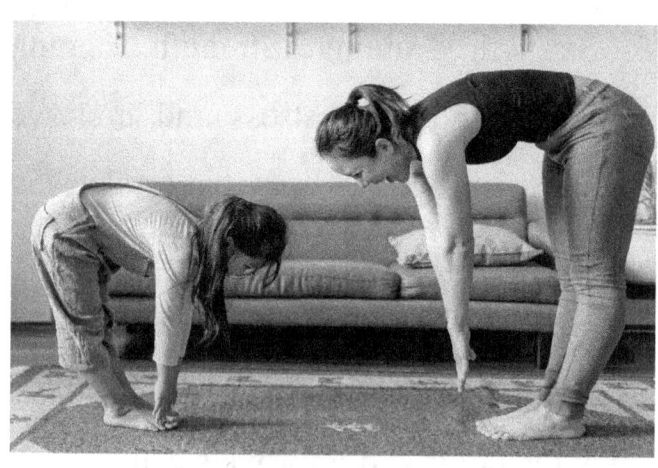

Promoting sleep through healthy diet

A healthy diet can promote sleep in a few ways. First, eating nutrient-dense foods that are high in fiber, vitamins, and minerals can help to regulate hormones which can improve sleep. Eating foods like lean proteins, complex carbohydrates, and healthy fats can help to keep blood sugar and energy levels balanced, which helps to maintain consistent sleep patterns.

Novel foods like vegetables, fruits, lean meats, and whole grains are also good sources of melatonin, a hormone that helps to regulate the body's sleep-wake cycle.

Eating foods that are high in magnesium and calcium, such as fish, dairy, and leafy greens, can also help to promote healthy sleep patterns, as these minerals are important for nerve and muscle relaxation.

In addition to eating healthy foods, avoiding processed foods and limiting stimulants like caffeine and sugar can also help to improve sleep. Eating a light snack before bed can also help to promote sleep, as it can help to regulate blood sugar levels and provide energy for the body to use while sleeping.

Finally, staying hydrated throughout the day can also help to promote sleep, as dehydration can disrupt sleep patterns.

Overall, eating a healthy diet can help to promote healthy sleep patterns by providing the body with the nutrients it needs to regulate hormones and energy levels, as well as support nerve and muscle relaxation. Eating healthy foods, avoiding processed foods and stimulants, eating a light snack before bed, and staying hydrated throughout the day are all great ways to promote healthy sleep.

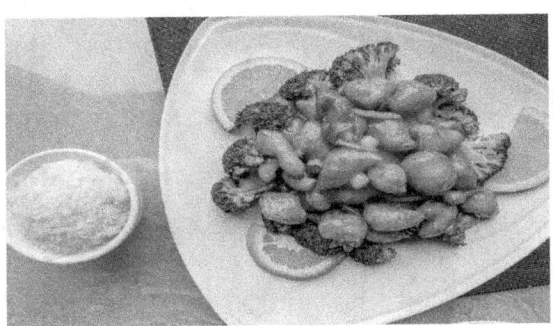

CHAPTER SIX

Insomnia-Prevention and Treatment Recipes

Foot Massage with Lavender

1 ounce (28g) of a carrier oil, such as olive, almond, jojoba, grape seed, or apricot.

12 drops of lavender essential oil (12 drops for children and pregnant women).

HOW TO PREPARE AND USE:

In a clean jar, pour the oil and lavender essential oil. Shake the cap.

Draw one foot onto your lap while you sit comfortably. One tablespoon (15 ml) of fragrant oil should be poured into your palm and massaged into your foot.

Give it some time. Swap the feet. If the night is cool, throw on some fresh socks. squirm into bed.

How it functions

It's comforting to use lavender. To reach the blood, the essential oil must pass through the skin.

When you breathe in the aroma, it also goes into your lungs. You can physically escape your busy mind by massaging your feet, which will aid in falling asleep. Inhaling a concoction of relaxing essential oils, including lavender, Roman chamomile, and neroli, reduced anxiety and enhanced sleep quality in cardiac patients in the intensive care unit, according to a 2013 study (a place notorious for disrupting sleep). The advantages are available to everyone. Inhaling lavender at night made healthy

Japanese students wake up feeling more rejuvenated, according to a research.

Alternative: Request that a lover or friend rub your feet (or back) for you. Try Roman chamomile, bergamot, rose geranium, melissa (lemon balm), neroli, jasmine, ylang ylang, and sandalwood, among other relaxing essential oils. It matters whether you find the perfume to be calming.

Tips

Have some chamomile tea. Since ancient times, the herb German chamomile has been used as a tea as a sleep aid. It contains sedative and anti-anxiety properties. In a group of chronic insomniacs receiving a chamomile extract, a preliminary investigation found a considerable improvement in daytime functioning but only modest advantages for sleep quantity and quality.

To prevent being awakened by a full bladder, drink tea at least an hour before going to bed.

Scented pillow for sleep

Lavender essential oil, 2 to 3 drops

SET UP AND USE: Place a clean pillowcase over your pillow. A few drops of lavender essential oil should be massaged into your palms. To spread the calming smell, rub your palms together and over the pillowcase.

How it works: Research demonstrates that the relaxing effects of lavender essential oil on the nervous system.

A research on menopausal women found that inhaling lavender enhanced their sleep quality (a change that frequently disturbs it).

Sleep-Promoting Sodium Bath

2 cups (480 g) (480 g) salts of epsom

10 drops of essential lavender oil

In a clean basin, combine the salts and lavender drops before using. Take a hot bath. Mix the ingredients together with your fingertips after adding them. Switch off the lights, please. Turn on a candle. Enter the fragrant, warm water. Relax. Crawl into bed once you go and towel off.

How it works: Being warm promotes relaxation and sleep. Likewise, violet. Another explanation is that taking a bath somewhat elevates your body temperature.

Your body temperature returns to normal after that. That decrease mimics the drop in body temperature that generally happens during sleep.

Magnesium sulfate makes up epsom salts. Unpublished research reveals that taking an Epsom salt bath can raise the amount of magnesium in the blood, which helps to calm tight muscles.

Tips

For you travelers, melatonin-containing tablets can aid with jet lag and other changes in daily rhythm. The majority of studies have employed doses between 2 and 8 milligrams, administered for up to three days prior to travel at a time that corresponds to bedtime at the destination. Additionally, travelers can use daylight to adjust to the new time zone. Your internal clock will advance due to early morning light (earlier awakening, earlier bedtime). Bright light later in the day causes your internal clock to change, causing you to rise and fall later. Supplements also appear to aid elderly adults with sleeplessness as melatonin levels decrease with age. Talk to your doctor about that choice.

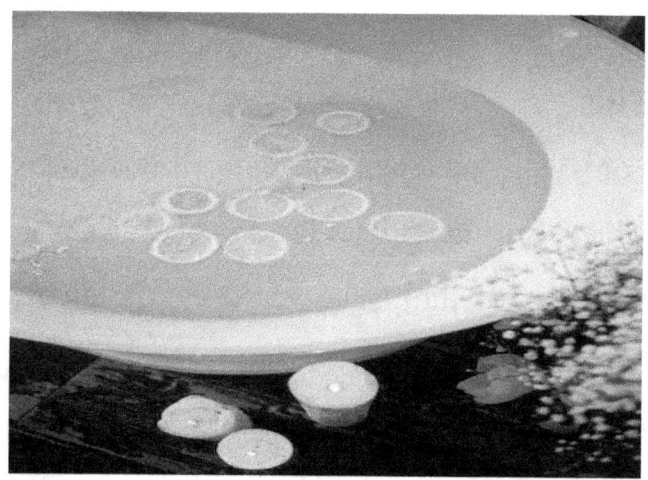

Purple Bath Bomb

221 g (1 cup) of baking soda

65 g (1/2 cup) of cornstarch

120 g or 1/2 cup of Epsom salts

12 cup (197 g) of citric acid powder (see note)

15 milliliters (15 tsp) of water

two teaspoons (10 ml) essential oil of lavender

15 ml of heated coconut oil or vegetable oil, one spoonful

HOW TO PREPARE AND USE:

All the dry ingredients should be combined in a sizable glass dish. until smooth, whisk.

Mix the liquids in a different, smaller glass dish (they will not blend perfectly).

Add the liquid gradually, about 1 teaspoon (5 ml) at a time, while continuing to whisk the dry ingredients. If you add the liquid too quickly, the ingredients will react. The end product should hold together in a clump and have a consistency similar to damp (not wet) sand.

Add another teaspoon (5 ml) of oil diluted with a teaspoon (5 ml) of water if the mixture is too dry. Add little amounts of cornstarch if it is too wet.

Halfway fill muffin tins by pressing into them. When dried, remove the bombs and place them in a jar with a secure lid. Put one bomb in a warm bath to relax.

How it functions: The bath's warmth calms and relaxes. The muscles are soothed by Epsom salts. Lavender has relaxing effects.

Note: Natural food stores, grocery stores, and craft supply shops all sell citric acid in powder form.

Stress Pad

Pen and paper

A pen

SET UP AND USE: Before you turn in for the night, jot down any issues that are bothering you. Say to yourself, "All of this can wait until the morning," when you've finished writing your list.

Write down any worries you have if you wake up throughout the night to help you forget about them.

How it functions

Relaxation in the present can be disrupted by plans for the future. You can get rid of your problems by writing them down. There are moments when the only worry is that you might forget to do something. If you put it in writing, you'll have a clear list of things to do the next day. Declare to yourself that you can let go now.

Tips

Consider your before-bed snacks. Oatmeal or a tiny slice of whole-grain toast may promote sleep. The carbs might assist in transferring the amino acid tryptophan from the blood into the brain, where it can undergo chemical reactions to become melatonin. A small snack can also stop blood sugar levels from falling too low at night.

Stress hormones are activated by low blood sugar, which may cause you to become awake. 'Light' is the key word here. A large late-night dinner can keep you awake.

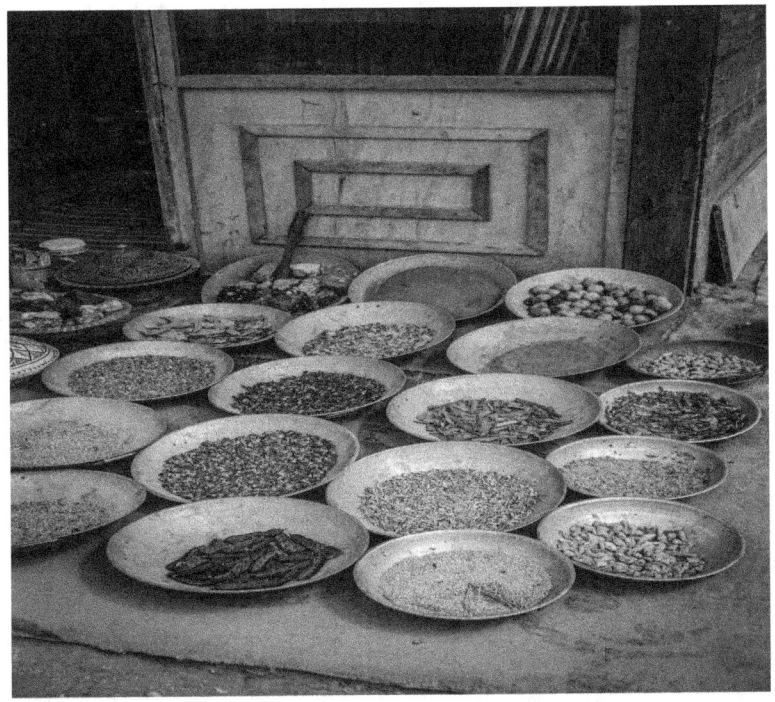

CHAPTER SEVEN

Retrain Your Brain (Stimulus Control Therapy)

Stimulus control therapy (SCT) is a form of therapy used to treat insomnia. SCT is based on the idea that certain environmental cues may be associated with sleep and that changing such cues can lead to better sleeping habits. It is typically used in combination with other forms of therapy, such as cognitive behavioral therapy (CBT).

The basic principle of SCT is to modify the environment to reduce cues that are associated with difficulty sleeping. This includes removing clocks or televisions from the bedroom, turning off lights and electronics, and avoiding caffeine or other substances that may interfere with sleep. Additionally, SCT encourages going to bed and waking up at the same time each day and avoiding naps.

Another important component of SCT is to associate the bed with sleep. This means that activities such as working, eating, or watching television in bed should be avoided. This can be difficult for some people, so it is important to find a comfortable chair or couch to use instead.

In addition to environmental changes, SCT may also involve cognitive restructuring. This involves changing how we think about sleep, such as by challenging negative thoughts about sleep and replacing them with positive ones. It is important to stick to the same schedule, even on weekends. It is also important to avoid napping during the day as this can disrupt the natural sleep-wake cycle. Additionally, SCT teaches the patient to use the bedroom only for sleeping. This means avoiding activities such as watching television, reading, eating, or working in the bedroom.

Another goal of SCT is to eliminate any negative associations the patient has with sleeping. This means avoiding worrying about sleep or dwelling on negative thoughts before going to bed. Instead, SCT encourages the patient to relax and use mental imagery or progressive muscle relaxation to help clear the mind. Additionally, SCT teaches the patient to get out of bed if they are unable to sleep and to not lay in bed worrying about sleep. The patient is encouraged to go to a different room and do a relaxing activity until they feel sleepy.

Let's consider a typical individual who is getting excellent sleep. Say she gets eight hours of sleep on average each night and enjoys reading in bed for about thirty minutes before her eyelids get too heavy to read.

She dims the lights and nods off right away. She sleeps soundly through the night, perhaps waking up only once to use the restroom for a brief period of time. She spends eight and a half hours in bed and rests for eight hours, or 94% of the time she is in bed.

As a result, her bed has a very powerful association with sleep in her brain. She can afford to do something else in bed (read) without disturbing her sleep, because over

90% of the time she is in bed, she is sleeping.

Her brain is aware that bed equals slumber on some unconscious level. Her brain begins to get ready for slumber when she gets into bed at night. How else could it function? Yes, the cot is for sleeping.

Now imagine that the same woman has gone through some stressful changes in her life and no longer falls asleep fast after turning out the lights. Instead, she starts to wonder, "Can I handle this new work position?" What if they decide that promoting me was an error? How will Tom and the kids react to my increased job schedule?

Melissa's academic struggles are getting progressively worse. How will I manage that when I have more work? Am I a terrible mother? I'm a poor mother. Like yesterday—why did I scream at Ryan? He wasn't really acting in a bad way.

As she attempts to sleep, her mind continues to race. Now, she only gets about six hours of slumber every night. She is worn out by evening, so she begins to go to bed earlier in an effort to get more sleep.

She spends nine hours in bed instead of eight and a half, and as time passes, nine and a half hours. However, she still only gets about six and a half hours of slumber per night. Currently, she spends only 68%, or two thirds, of the time in bed asleep.

She doesn't just read and sleep in bed; she also worries while conscious. Sleep no longer equates to bed. A bed is a place to study, worry, or simply doze off. Her brain does not immediately begin the sleep-preparation process when she gets into bed at night. the reason why? Instead of sleeping, it might be time to read, worry, or simply lay there. Her slumber issues might worsen over time.

Her thoughts might be awakened when she returns to bed after getting up in the middle of the night to use the restroom. She now experiences prolonged awakenings in the midst of the night in addition to difficulty falling asleep in the morning.

The program called stimulus control therapy (SCT) can help you retrain your brain to firmly associate sleeping in bed with falling asleep. In order to achieve this, we must reduce the connection between bed and all other activities, including internal states of arousal and other activities (like reading or viewing television) (such as frustration, stress, fear, or worry).

When you go to bed, you should limit the choices available to your brain and body. We also want to lessen the link between sleeping in places other than your room. In other words, you will only slumber in your bed and use it for those purposes. We know that SCT works both from our clinical experience and from well-controlled research studies. SCT was the first behavioral program designed to treat insomnia.

For whom is Stimulus Control Treatment Appropriate?

Both stimulus control and sleep restriction are likely to be effective for you, so we typically advise choosing the one that you are most motivated to completely implement. Nevertheless, depending on your sleep pattern, one treatment might suit you better on occasion. Here are some clues that SCT is likely to perform well for you:

• Your insomnia manifests as protracted periods of vigilance at the start, middle, or conclusion of the night.

• You use your bed or bedroom for purposes other than sex and slumber, such as when you are unable to fall asleep.

• You don't just slumber in your bed (such as a couch or a guest room).

• You fall asleep while you are in another room, but when you get into bed, you feel more aware or anxious.

• When you're not at home, you slumber better. If any of the following apply to your sleep: • Your slumber is fragmented, restless, or unrefreshing, but you are not consistently awake.

- Throughout the night, you experience numerous brief (but not protracted) awakenings.
- You take medication or have a medical condition that makes getting out of bed in the middle of the night risky or challenging for you.

Treatment for Sensory Control

1. Restrict activities in bed and your bedroom to sex and sleep.

Remember, we want the bed to cue your brain to slumber, and only sleep. What else do you do in your bed or boudoir, take stock? Watch any TV? use a PC, tablet, or smartphone? Read? Do you and your bed companion talk? Do you obsessively think about the past while you're lying in bed? Or do you worry, make plans, try to solve problems, or indulge in fantasies?

If any of these questions were yes, find a place other than your bedroom where you can carry out these tasks. Give your electronic devices a fresh "home."

Decide where you will study, write, or pay bills in another room. Why is intimacy permitted but not other things? The majority of us, according to Bootzin and Perlis (2011, 24), "just aren't very creative about where we have intercourse"!

2. Only lie down if you're tired.

This is a little trickier than it appears. You should go to bed when you are tired to increase your chances of falling asleep fast (remember, the goal is for bed to equal sleep). A regular bedtime, though, does assist. Therefore, we advise choosing a target bedtime and preparing yourself to feel sleepy by that time each night by beginning to wind down about 60 minutes early and going through your bedtime rituals (like shaving and donning pajamas) as though you were going to go to bed at your target time.

Get into bed and put out the lights if you're tired. If you're not tired, avoid the bedroom and engage in activities that will make you feel drowsy; then, when you are, retire to bed.

This rule does not apply to everyone because some people do not become sleepy until they lay down in a dark environment. If this sounds like you, you can experiment by going to bed at your goal bedtime each night, regardless of how sleepy you are. You will get up if you don't fall unconscious in about twenty minutes (see step 3).

3. If you are awake for more than twenty minutes at any point during the night, get out of bed and do something uninteresting or soothing.

According to the initial SCT guidelines, you should get out of bed if you are awake for ten minutes. To try to find a balance, we advise that you exit the bedroom after twenty minutes.

On the one hand, we need to cut down on the quantity of time you spend awake in bed. On the other hand, we don't want to build up irrational expectations because it is entirely normal for it to take up to twenty minutes to fall asleep.

Given our primary goal of retraining your brain, you can absolutely get up sooner if you are so annoyed, or anxious that you know sleep isn't coming anytime soon.

Here are a few more suggestions.

• Check the time when you have a strong feeling of it rather than keeping an eye on the clock.

It's been around 20 minutes. With experience, your estimation skills will improve.

• Make a plan. Plan your route and your next steps. Prepare your tools.

Utilize dim illumination. If you are reading on a computer with backlighting, dim it as much as you can and turn off any other lights.

Use a light with a low-wattage (about 25 watts) bulb instead. Your brain receives a signal from darkness that it is nightfall; light is stimulating. Because of the light that screens produce, some people advise against using anything with a screen (phone, electronic reader, computer). If you are not willing to avoid screens, consider wearing sunglasses that block out the blue \srays of the light spectrum. On the Internet, these are easily accessible for purchase.

• Select monotonous or calming pursuits over stimulating ones, such as folding laundry, ironing, knitting, reading, or listening to podcasts or audiobooks. Choose items you can set down at any moment (such as uncomplicated knitting projects, magazines with short articles, books you have read before). If you decide to read or listen to something, choose something that won't overly stimulate your thoughts.

Everyone has a varied ability to do this; some can read or listen to the news while others become too anxious; some people can read or listen to work-related material while others cannot.

• Pick tasks that don't require a lot of productivity from you. You don't want to spend so much time reading or doing chores that your brain starts to believe that nights are the best time for work.

• Foresee problems and find solutions. For example, if it will be hard to get out of bed because the house will be cold, have a bathrobe and slippers beside \syour bed and a blanket where you will be sitting. Have water ready for you if you know you'll be thirsty and the kitchen is up a flight of steps.

4. Go back to bed when you're tired. (Don't go to bed in a different area.)

There is no set period of time for getting out of bed. Before your rise time, you might experience sleepiness and go back to bed in a matter of minutes, or it might take hours. Return to bed as soon as you start to feel sleepy and allow yourself up to 20 minutes to nod off.

There is one exception, just like retiring to bed early in the evening.

Remember, part of strengthening the link between bed and sleep is to sleep only in bed. Therefore, even if going to your bedroom makes you feel more alert, SCT will function best in the long run if you don't doze off somewhere else.

5. Repeat steps 3-4 as needed.

You might get up and go back to bed several times, just once, or not at all on any particular night.

6. Establish a wake time that you adhere to every morning, regardless of how much sleep you received.

We frequently advise having a regular wake time if you are only ready to make one change to improve your sleep. This step's significance cannot be emphasized!

By adjusting your wake time, you can develop a regular sleep-wake rhythm that promotes sound slumber and reduces daytime sleepiness. Also, if you stay in bed later some mornings, fewer hours will have passed and your sleep drive will be \slower at your target bedtime the next night, possibly making it harder to fall asleep quickly.

On days off from work, you are allowed to "sleep in" for up to an hour longer, according to the standard SCT instructions. Generally speaking, we advise against doing this so you can benefit fully from a regular sleep-wake cycle. If you have to get up earlier than your natural wake-up time on workdays and are getting substantially less sleep than you need, we are more likely to support a later rising time on non-workdays (as opposed to scrounging up the necessary amount of sleep, but in an erratic manner). In these situations, sleeping an additional hour two mornings a week can help you feel less tired, and your overall "sleep debt" will make it easier for you to fall asleep at your intended bedtime even if you slept in.

If you attempt to stay up later on days off from work and discover that you sleep worse the following night, we advise having a regular wake time every day.

We advise you to choose times that give you a "sleep window" of no more than the total amount of sleep you believe you require each night when choosing your goal bedtime and regular wake-up time. If you need eight hours of sleep, for instance, pick 10:30 p.m.–6:30 a.m. rather than 9:30 p.m.–7 a.m. It is normal for you to allow yourself a longer window of time to sleep because you have grown accustomed to being awake in the middle of the night. However, as you will see if you learn about sleep deprivation or the application of SCT and SRT together, this frequently backfires. No rests during the day.

Naps prevent you from taking advantage of the ability of sleep deprivation to assist you in falling asleep fast and staying asleep at night.

Additionally, sleeping during the day might make it harder for you to associate slumber with the night, which is something you want to do. Last but not least, most people do not take their naps in their bedrooms during the day. Keep in mind that you should only slumber in beds to strengthen the connection between bed and sleep.

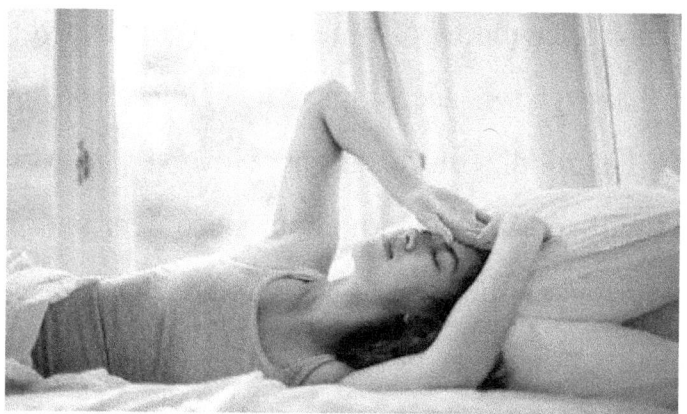

Typical Queries (and Answers) and How to Prepare

How long will it take for this therapy to be effective?

Your ability to sleep may improve almost immediately once you realize that there is a plan and you won't be forced to spend hours in bed awake. This relief will likely result in less physical arousal and better sleep. For some individuals, the power of the plan itself is sufficient; they hardly ever leave their beds. Or you might see fast progress just from taking back the hours of your life that you had lost to insomnia. Even if you are not getting more sleep, you might feel a lot better by getting out of bed and spending more time engaging in pleasant activities.

However, for the majority of people, improvement requires more time. Your memory may need to be retrained for a few weeks. You will be getting used to a new routine the first few evenings, and you may even feel a little anxious about the treatment, which could make it difficult for you to fall asleep. People frequently call us at this juncture looking for assurance.

Our general response is that it is normal to be anxious or worried, and we have very high confidence that the program will work if you do it completely and persist with it. In this manner, we also want to inspire you. Additionally, you might originally feel worse because you might actually get less sleep. Let's assume that after getting out of bed because you couldn't sleep for 30 minutes, you went back to bed.

If you had remained in bed, you might have fallen asleep in just five minutes, in which case performing SCT would have cost you twenty-five minutes of sleep.

Do you already feel nervous after reading this?

When you are dealing with persistent insomnia, we understand how difficult it can be to sacrifice valuable sleep time. Keep in mind that the reason you are reading this book is because what you are doing right now is ineffective.

Are you willing to put up with more now in order to obtain more later?

We do not state this in jest. We are aware of the difficulties. We are asking you to put in this difficult work because we have witnessed the dramatic change in people who have endured the discomfort of insomnia for years or even decades when they were prepared to initially feel even worse.

Your progress might not be linear, regardless of how fast you improve or how long it takes.

"Take two strides forward and one step back" is acceptable. Attempt this exercise: get up, and choose a spot about ten feet away. Take two strides in the direction you want to go, then one step in the opposite direction. Where do you wind up doing this if you keep doing it? If you keep going, even though it might take longer and require more effort than moving forward continuously, you will eventually arrive at your goal.

What you do after a loss depends entirely on how you handle it. You will cause more physical arousal and find it more difficult to fall asleep again that night or the next morning if you react with dread or utter frustration.

You might also decide to stop using the therapy altogether. This response to what might have been a brief loss can leave you exactly where you were before. On the other hand, there is a good chance the backward step will be followed by another two forward if you can maintain the program and exercise acceptance and surrender to whatever this evening brings.

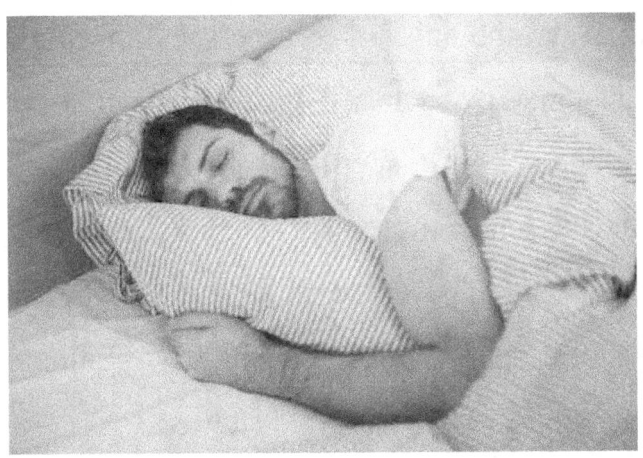

CHAPTER EIGHT

(Sleep Restriction Treatment) Quality Over Quantity

Sleep restriction therapy is a form of cognitive behavioral therapy (CBT) used to treat insomnia. It involves reducing the amount of time spent in bed in order to increase the amount of time spent sleeping. This therapy is based on the idea that the amount of time spent in bed should match the amount of time spent sleeping.

The goal of sleep restriction therapy is to restore healthy sleep patterns by re-training the body to fall asleep and stay asleep.

It can be done in combination with other therapies such as cognitive behavioral therapy, relaxation training, and stimulus control.

The first step in sleep restriction therapy is to determine the amount of time it takes to get to sleep. This is usually done by keeping a sleep log for one to two weeks. This log will record how long it takes to get to sleep and how long you stay asleep.

Once the amount of time it takes to get to sleep is determined, the next step is to reduce the amount of time spent in bed. This is done by setting a strict bedtime and rising time and sticking to it. This will ensure that the amount of time spent in bed matches the amount of time spent sleeping.

During the sleep restriction period, it is important to practice good sleep hygiene such as avoiding caffeine and alcohol in the evening, keeping the bedroom dark and quiet, and avoiding screens before bed. Avoiding napping during the day is also important.

The amount of time spent in bed can be increased gradually as the sleep improves. This will help to maintain the improved sleep pattern.

As an effective treatment for insomnia, sleep restriction therapy can help to restore healthy sleep patterns and improve overall sleep quality. It is important to remember that this therapy is not a quick fix, and it may take several weeks or months to see the full effects.

Spending more and more time "trying" to fall asleep is a typical reaction to unreliable slumber. You might continue to spend more time in bed. Or perhaps there are longer intervals between your original bedtime and final rise time, with periods spent awake.

Or maybe you snooze during the day. Getting more slumber might be your goal every night of the week or just on the weekends. Your sleep spreads out to fill the larger area you give it as you spend more time attempting to fall asleep.

If you typically get six hours of sleep, for instance, you might object, "Yeah, but they're not even six decent hours!"

In sleep restriction therapy (SRT), we reduce your sleep window (the hours you designate for sleeping) to a level that is consistent with the amount of sleep your body is presently receiving. The outcome? Your slumber is probably going to knit back together and have fewer interruptions, which will make it deeper and more restful. Because you won't be receiving enough sleep at first, you may still experience all the daytime effects of insomnia, such as fatigue or "foggy" thinking. But once you've established a solid foundation of consolidated sleep, we'll expand on it to help you return to a healthy level of sleep.

Who is Sleep Restriction Therapy meant for?

Both sleep restriction and stimulus control are likely to be effective for you, so we frequently advise choosing the strategy that you are most motivated to completely implement.

Having said that, if any of the following holds true, we would advise SRT over SCT:

• You have sporadic, restless, or unrefreshing slumber but are occasionally partially awake.

• Throughout the night, you experience numerous brief (but not protracted) awakenings.

• Mobility problems prevent you from performing SCT because it is risky to get out of bed when you are not asleep.

If you presently have some nights of adequate sleep and are unwilling to give these up, we advise starting with SCT rather than SRT.

• Even after reading about this obstacle later in this chapter, you are unwilling to limit the amount of time you spend in bed.

Detailed Directions for Sleep Restriction Therapy

Now let's look carefully at each step. Although the steps may appear straightforward in theory, clients frequently have a lot of concerns once they begin to consider actually completing the program.

1. Using the data from your sleep log for ten to fourteen days, determine your average total sleep time (TST), average time in bed (TIB), and sleep efficiency (SE). Continue if SE is greater than 90% (or 85% for older people).

The percentage of time you spend sleeping in bed is your sleep effectiveness. Prior to falling asleep at the start of the night, the majority of individuals do stay awake for ten to twenty minutes.

Additionally, having one or two brief awakenings is entirely normal (depending on your age and other factors). So, we don't anticipate a perfect efficacy. Since individuals do experience more awakenings as they get older, 90% for youth and adults and 85% for older adults is a good target.

Even if your average SE is higher than 90%, there are instances when SRT should be used. This will raise your average, for instance, if your SE was high only on the evenings you used sleeping pills.

Only the evenings when you did not use a sleep aid can be used to determine your average total amount of sleep. The original SRT prescription that is written for you is based on this.

Additionally, SRT can definitely be effective if your technical SE is over 90% due to the fact that you do not remain in bed when you are not asleep but are asleep less than 90% of the time between your initial bedtime and final rise time.

2. Do not spend less than five hours in bed, but no less than your average TST. Set a regular bedtime and wake-up hour to achieve this.

To find your present average TST, keep in mind that it's best to use data from ten to fourteen nights of sleep tracking. You should set your TIB equal to your average TST if you are presently sleeping more than five hours per night on average. You'll set your TIB to five hours if not.

The creators of this treatment originally recommended a lower limit of four hours and thirty minutes for prescribed TIB, but they increased this to five hours because less than that caused too much sleep deprivation at the start of treatment and didn't provide enough additional benefit to justify this cost.

How do you choose which hours to sleep once you've determined the number of hours you'll be in bed?

There are various approaches to this. We tend to agree with the SRT creators in that we advise scheduling your sleep window for the portion of the night that is most likely to include your best slumber. For example, if you fall asleep easily and get several hours of solid sleep before waking up, start \syour sleep window at your desired bedtime. Set your sleep window for the later part of the night and wake up at your preferred rise time if, on the other hand, the early hours of the night are the hardest and you eventually fall asleep deeply at 3 a.m.

Reduce the amount of time spent in bed at both ends if the middle part of the night provides the most peaceful sleep. Consider what schedule will be most convenient for you if there is no recognizable trend or if your sleep is inconsistent throughout the entire night.

Is it easier to picture getting up early or staying up later?

If, after taking all of this into account, you are still unsure, our default is to have you stay up longer and get up when you want to. We make this claim for two reasons: (1) most of our clients report that forcing themselves to stay up later is easier than forcing themselves out of bed before sunrise; and (2) having a fixed wake time is one of the best anchors for your internal clock, and if you start with it at your desired rise time, you won't need to adjust it throughout the treatment program.

The time you intend to go to bed once your slumber has stabilized is referred to as your "desired bedtime." Start your sleep window no earlier than 10:30 p.m. if you would normally aim for 10:30 p.m.-6 a.m. but have been going to bed at 9 p.m. because you're so tired. We refer to your "desired rise time" as the earliest time you must awaken in order to fulfill your obligations (child care, job, school), as opposed to your ideal wake-up time (worship services, running group). Therefore, set your wake-up time to no later than 6:30 if you need to get up by 6:30 twice per week. One crucial aspect of SRT is maintaining a consistent sleep-wake routine, not just a constrained one.

3. No afternoon naps.

Your sleep urge will be reduced even by quick naps. We are not positive, but even tiny "nod offs" close to bed may make a big difference in some people's sleep drive. A stronger sleep drive will help you fall asleep quickly and remain asleep throughout the night.

4. Adjust your bedtime: Increase your TIB by fifteen minutes when your average SE over a one-week period is 90% (85% for older adults). Reduce your TIB to your current average TST, but not less than five hours, if your one-week average SE is less than 85% (80% for older people). Make no changes if your SE is 85%–89% (or 80%–84% for older people).

Maintaining your sleep diary is crucial while performing SRT. This will not only enable you to assess your level of program compliance honestly, but it will also give you the data you require to determine when it is appropriate to lengthen (or shorten) your bedtime. You'll notice that in this command, your TIB is being changed based on data from the entire past week, not just from one particular night.

This will enable you to create the strong foundation of consolidated sleep that we are looking for, guard against "kneejerk" reactions to one particularly "good" or "bad" night, and possibly prevent you from placing undue strain on yourself to sleep on any given night.

A "one-week interval" is any stretch of seven days that follow each other, not just a week in the calendar. You are welcome to compute your averages once a week, or more frequently using the information from the preceding seven nights. Say, for instance, that during the first week of treatment, your SE is 88% (causing you to maintain your TIB) and that the last four nights have been obviously better than the first three.

You might want to check to see if your SE has met the 90% benchmark after three more days on the program rather than waiting another seven nights. Instead of waiting the full two weeks, you can raise your TIB after ten nights if your seven-day average SE is currently 90%.

If their original prescription was set at their current average TST, our clients very rarely need to reduce their TIB. Theoretically, it is possible that during the program, your sleep will become even less effective and that your SE will drop into the region where it is advised that you reduce TIB.

However, we have only had this happen with clients who began with a more gentle restriction, and therefore could not really expect to sleep 85% of the time they were in bed.

5. Keep going back to step 4 until you get the recommended amount of sleep.

Consider your goal as the quantity of sleep that will leave you feeling rested and able to function well during the day. Nobody's standard will fit everyone's needs. Your own slumber requirements may even alter over time.

Through this training, you might learn that you require less sleep than you initially believed. For instance, you might believe right now that you work best with eight hours. Consider adding fifteen minutes of TIB each week while still reaching the 90% SE mark in the first six weeks of treatment. The SE drops below 85% in week 7 as you raise TIB to seven and a half hours and experience some sleep fragmentation. You make the choice to go back to seven and a quarter hours TIB because you feel rested and there won't be any problems during the day. This would be a triumph, and we would rejoice.

The objective of treatment is to help you get the sleep you truly need, not just the amount of sleep you think you need. You shouldn't live to slumber; rather, you should sleep to live. A major part of this is concentrating on how you feel during the day rather than how much sleep you get at night.

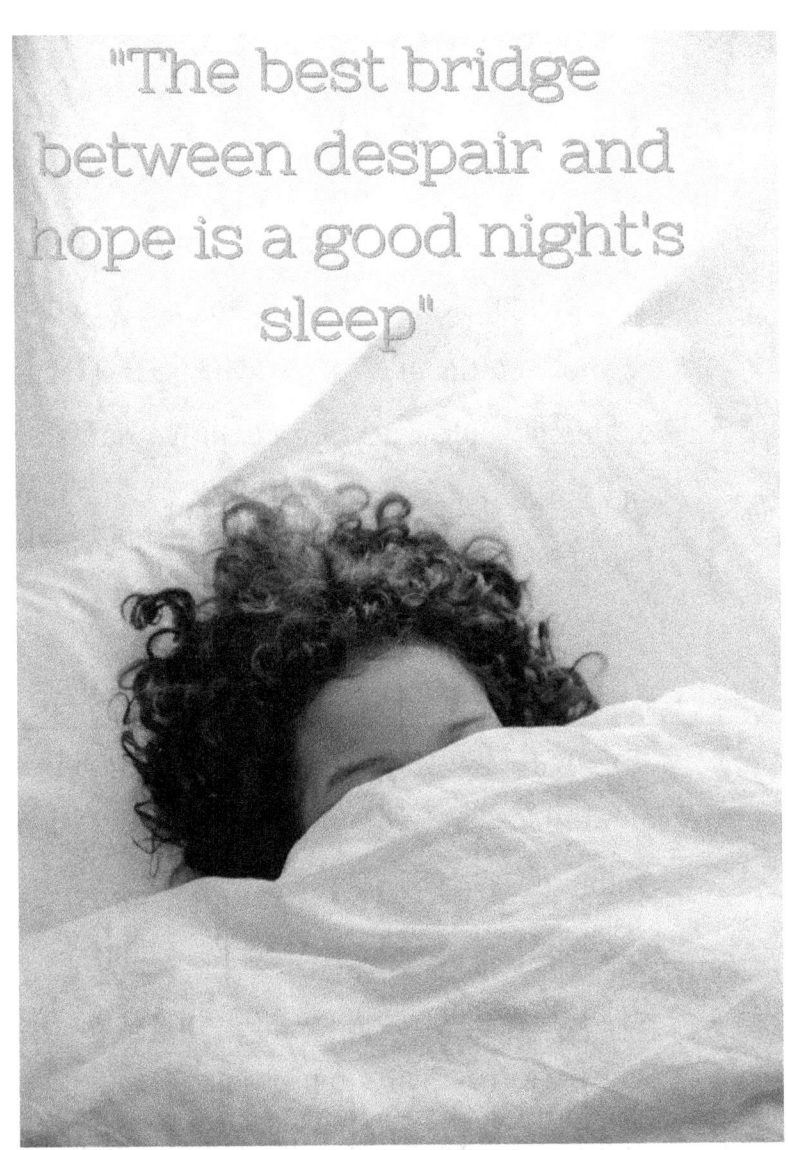

"The best bridge between despair and hope is a good night's sleep"

CHAPTER NINE

Mental Health and Sleep

Numerous mental exercise techniques exist. Two mental skills that we have discovered to be most pertinent to sleep will be the focus of this chapter. They are cognitive defusion and mindfulness.

Poor sleepers who use these techniques have been able to improve their capacity for restful, rejuvenating slumber. Anywhere, at any moment, is a good place to practice mindfulness and cognitive defusion techniques.

You can perform them officially using tools like pillows and guided recordings, or you can perform them impromptu using only your thoughts and your breath. Guided audio recordings are included in this book to help you practice these abilities.

Mindfulness

Intentional attention to the present moment is mindfulness. When you are "full of thought," that is. It alludes to any instance in which you consciously decide to focus on what is taking place right now.

Let's attempt an illustration. Set a thirty-second stopwatch. During those thirty seconds, challenge yourself to listen carefully to the noises all around you. You can perform this while keeping your eyes open or closed and in any relaxed posture. Just make an effort to deliberately pay attention to the noises around you. When the time has past, pose the following queries to yourself.

This is an illustration of awareness instruction. To be completely present in this instant, you engaged in a deliberate and focused exercise. You directed your attention in this exercise using one of your five senses.

You noted how your attention changed (or not). You also took note of any ideas that surfaced, if any. Since there isn't really a right or wrong method to practice mindfulness, there's no need to evaluate how well you performed this mindful exercise. To give attention to your attention is all that is necessary.

According to studies, our brains can change in as little as eight weeks with a daily mindfulness exercise that lasts a total of about thirty minutes.

Achieving a condition of happiness, contentment, or a clear mind is not the goal of mindfulness. When we focus on the present instant, we frequently learn painful or unpleasant things.

Being mindful involves using your attention and concentration to be as receptive as you can to the experiences you are having in this very moment. Being mindful means paying attention to your thoughts, emotions, and sensations as they arise.

You can develop your capacity to observe whatever arises, without necessarily having to react to it, through awareness training. This can support you in achieving your objectives. For instance, mindfulness can be beneficial when you become aware of your worrying ideas regarding your sleep schedule.

Despite these concerns, you can continue with the program because it supports your desire to get better slumber.

The word "mindfulness" may also conjure images of meditation in your head. Information on the parallels and differences between these two ideas is widely available. We'll use the term "mindfulness" to describe the deliberate act of focusing on the present instant for our purposes. We will refer to a particular kind of "formal" mindfulness exercise as "meditation." We don't want you to stress out too much about these markings, though. Whatever you want to name it, improving your capacity for intentional focus and attention is incredibly beneficial for sleep. This is due to the fact that you are educating your mind to maintain contact with the current. If your thinking is keeping you awake, you can use this to calm it down. It will also enable you to recognize anxious or arousal-inducing ideas and handle them coolly. Try exercising for five or ten minutes if you find this thirty-second exercise to be helpful.

Activities for Mindfulness

Focusing on the present moment while acknowledging and accepting one's feelings, thoughts, and physical sensations constitutes the psychological practice of mindfulness. It is a powerful tool for managing stress, improving mental health, and developing a greater sense of well-being. There are a variety of activities that can be used to practice mindfulness, from simple breathing exercises to more complex meditations.

Some of the most popular mindfulness activities include

1. Meditation: Meditation is the most common form of mindfulness practice. It involves sitting quietly and focusing on your breath, allowing thoughts and feelings to come and go without judgment. Over time, this practice can help to increase awareness and reduce stress.

2. Body Scanning: Body scanning is a type of meditation that involves focusing on different parts of the body in order to become aware of sensations and any tightness or tension. It is a great tool for relaxation and can help to reduce stress and anxiety.

3. Mindful Eating: Mindful eating involves paying attention to the experience of eating, rather than engaging in other activities while

eating. This includes focusing on the flavors, textures, and smells of the food, as well as noticing how the body responds to the food.

4. Mindful Movement: Mindful movement is any type of exercise that is done with awareness and attention. This could be yoga, tai chi, walking, or any other type of physical activity. It is important to focus on the sensations in the body while doing the activity and to be aware of the thoughts and feelings that come up.

5. Gratitude Practice: Gratitude practice is a way to cultivate appreciation for the present moment and all the good things in life. It involves taking time to reflect on what you are grateful for and to express appreciation for them.

6. Creative Expression: Creative expression is any type of activity that allows you to express yourself, such as writing, drawing, painting, photography, or any other form of art. It is a great way to tap into your emotions and connect to yourself.

7. Nature Walks: Nature walks can be a great way to practice mindfulness. Take time to observe your surroundings, noticing the sights, sounds, and smells of nature. Allow yourself to be present in the moment and be aware of any thoughts or feelings that come up.

These are just a few of the activities that can be used to practice mindfulness. Whatever activity you choose, it is important to be kind and compassionate with yourself, and to allow yourself to be present with whatever comes up.

Cognitive Defusion

Our second mental fitness aid, cognitive defusion, is derived from A&C therapy (ACT). Cognitive Defusion is a technique that has been found to be useful in treating insomnia. It seeks to help people identify and manage their thoughts and beliefs about sleep, and to challenge any negative thoughts that may be preventing them from getting a restful night's sleep.

The basic concept of cognitive defusion is to recognize that thoughts are just thoughts, and to not become entangled in their content. The goal is to take a step back from the thought and look at it from a more objective perspective. This helps to reduce the emotional intensity of the thought and its power to interfere with sleep.

For people with insomnia, cognitive defusion can help to reduce the anxiety and worry that often accompany thoughts about not being able to sleep. It can also help to break the cycle of rumination and worrying that can become a major obstacle to getting a good night's rest.

In practical terms, cognitive defusion involves identifying and labeling thoughts as they arise, and then changing the way they are perceived. For example, one might label a thought as "worrying" and then recall that worries are just thoughts, not facts. Once this is recognized, the thought can be observed and accepted, rather than fought against.

Another way to approach cognitive defusion is to recognize the thought, but then reframe it in a more positive light. For example, instead of "I can't sleep," one could reframe the thought to "I'm doing my best to get a good night's sleep." This helps to reduce the intensity of the thought and to adopt a more accepting attitude.

We also miss out on additional, frequently beneficial knowledge. Consider a camera's telescopic lens as an example. When you zoom in, only a tiny portion of the image is in focus. Everything else is blocked out by your telescopic lens. Imagine that your eye and the lens have merged together. You are no longer a subject being observed by a telescope.

The focus is you. You are both that lens and you as an individual simultaneously. Fusion is that.

Note that fusion is not inherently evil. Union can be useful in some circumstances. Being attentive is essential when traveling in traffic. You want to focus all of your attention and ideas on driving. Distractions such as the radio or your phone should be disregarded. Fusion, however, is frequently ineffective in circumstances involving sleep. Zooming in on the experience while attempting to sleep can be challenging. Your worries are amplified by the zoom lens. You enter the insomnia spiral when you become completely consumed by your emotions at these times.

You can learn the ability of cognitive defusion, which enables you to take a step back from the ideas your mind is producing. In defusion, we are more concerned with how to switch to a wide-angle lens rather than whether the claims are true. This has to do with how you and your ideas interact. You can help yourself and your mind become more objective and less emotional by "defusing" yourself from the thoughts that are going through your head.

Activities for Cognitive Difficulty

Cognitive defusion can be practiced in a variety of methods. Exercises that focus on the senses are crucial, just like with awareness. Although contemplating and reading about defusion is beneficial, it won't necessarily increase your cerebral stamina. Here are some practical starting point suggestions.

Use a name to control it. Consider one or two of your most upsetting sleep-related ideas. Repeat them several times to yourself. Right now, jot them down on paper. The paper should be placed on the ground about two feet in front of you. Hear these ideas out loud.

Now read them once more while circling the sheet of paper. Keep these ideas in mind as you move away from the paper.

What have you observed? You may have thought, Oh no, not that one again; it keeps coming up like a busted record. You might have also thought to yourself: I ponder why I am doing this as I stand over these thoughts. Whatever you may have thought, you most likely gained a sense of who you are as a person, independent of these ideas. You are who you are, and those written lines represent your ideas. Your ideas do not make you. Whatever the defusion is that display on the TV. Consider the television shows that offer ongoing information, such as the news, sports networks, and weather stations.

A continuous flood of words scrolls across the bottom of the television ticker. The data at the bottom of the screen simply continues appearing. It can be brand-new knowledge occasionally or outdated information being repeated. There is frequently concurrent writing happening elsewhere.

Now picture your ideas as the information displayed in the ticker at the bottom of the screen. The individual watching this data scroll across the screen is you. Sometimes it contains fresh data. It frequently just recounts a narrative. You are engaging in cognitive defusion when you become aware of your presence here and the presence of your ideas there (on the screen).

Make fun of the "packing." Playing with ideas' form is another strategy for calming them down. There are numerous options for doing this.

Proclaim your ideas out loud! Put them in an operatic style, or set them to the beat of a well-known music or jingle. Write an idea down on the computer screen. Put each repetition in a different typeface size and style after you've copied it several times.

• You can keep in mind that thoughts are just that—thoughts by engaging in any of these activities.

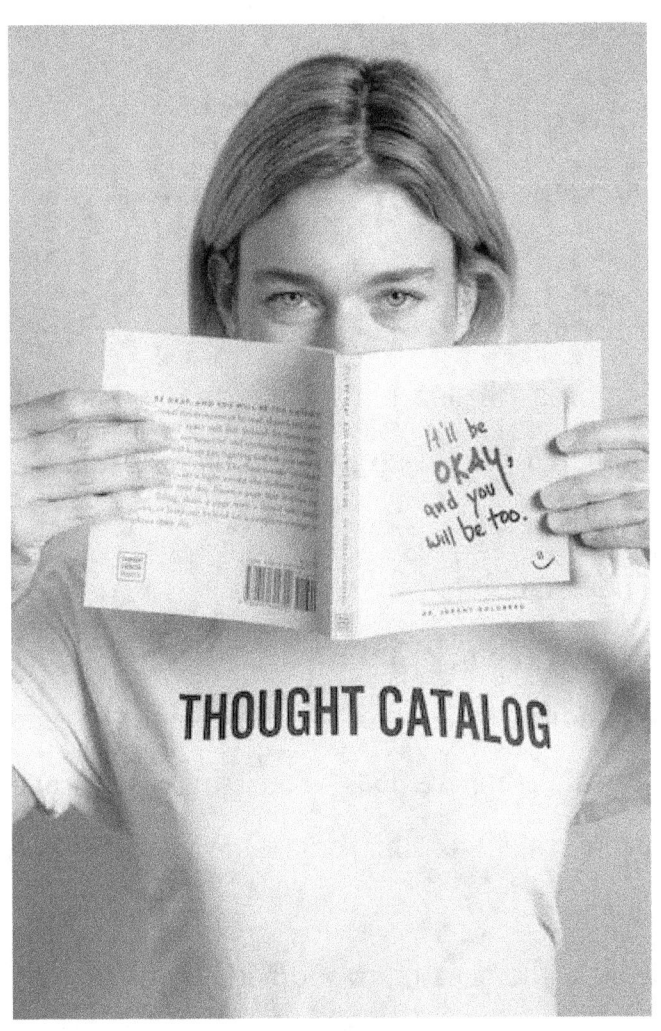

CHAPTER TEN

Thinking Differently (Cognitive Remodeling)

Humans are considered to generate hundreds, if not thousands, of thoughts each hour. This mind-boggling quantity of data is intended to aid in your quest for understanding.

Many things influence our thoughts, including our views, expectations, and personal experiences. Your mind sorts and arranges all of this data using groups and labels.

Using themes like good/bad, always/never, right/wrong, and love/hate, your mind organizes your ideas. Now tune into your thoughts. What do you believe? Maybe you're starting to feel curious about this chapter. Perhaps you're reflecting on your last night's sleep. Try to remember how your subconscious organized these thoughts. You might have described your curiosity as "useful" and your slumber from the previous night as "problematic." Give your ideas some thought for a moment or two.

Thoughts are not entirely reliable. They don't just generate positive ideas, either. When people are tired or experiencing strong emotions, their minds are frequently even less reliable and useful.

For instance, you might be more likely to think, "I'm never going to sleep tonight," if you're tired and worried about your slumber. Of course, this idea only fuels the cycle of insomnia. You have a negative emotional response, like frustration or despair. Your nervous system is then alerted by these feelings that something is amiss. Your body receives a signal from this to become more alert so it can deal with the problematic circumstance. Of course, this makes it more difficult to slumber.

For whom Should Cognitive Restructuring Be Used?

Cognitive restructuring (CR) can assist you in overcoming misconceptions about what "normal" sleep entails, dire predictions of what will happen if you don't get enough rest, unfavorable thoughts about other aspects of your life that cause stress or anxiety, and beliefs that limit your willingness to make changes to your sleep-related behaviors.

The following are some indicators that brain restructuring will probably benefit you:

• You tend to think in terms of "should" or "must," such as: I should be able to fall slumber within five minutes, I must sleep tonight, or I should sleep uninterruptedly through the night.

• Your health or ability to operate may be negatively impacted by your insomnia.

• Your ideas about sleeping are intrusive or anxious.

• You believe that your sleep issues are made worse by worry, anxiety, or depression.

• You think it's impossible for you to alter a behavior that you know would be beneficial.

• You don't think using behavioral techniques to treat your sleeplessness will work.

Bad Thoughts

Negative cognitions are distorted or unproductive ideas (or both). Your body is activated by negative thoughts, which mess with your sleep and wake patterns.

Bad thoughts also make you feel more uncomfortable. They increase the likelihood that you'll opt for temporary sleep remedies. They decrease your likelihood of making decisions that promote long-term, sustainable sleep habits. They interfere with your slumber, which is disruptive.

They fuel the cycle of your sleeplessness.

You should be aware of these three factors regarding negative thoughts. First of all, having unfavorable ideas about your sleep is common. It's very human to react negatively to a difficult circumstance.

Second, when you're tired or experiencing strong feelings, you're more likely to think negatively. Most individuals who battle with sleep have lots of negative thoughts about sleep.

Thirdly, unfavorable ideas breed unfavorable thoughts. Once a negative idea surfaces, more negative ones will follow. Negative emotions are therefore normal, but they can also cause you to have insomnia. Because they help you remove distortions and replace them with more accurate ideas, cognitive strategies are a crucial component of cognitive behavioral therapy (CBT).

CONCLUSION

The path to conquering insomnia can be a difficult one, but one that is worth the effort. By making a commitment to understanding your sleep needs, finding solutions that work for your lifestyle, and taking steps to improve your sleep environment and routine, you can learn to take control of your sleeping patterns and reclaim your nights.

You have learned everything from the science behind insomnia to the different treatments and strategies to deal with it. You have learned why certain behaviors and thoughts can cause or worsen insomnia, and what strategies you can use to take control of your sleep. You now have the knowledge and the tools to manage your own sleep problems.

No matter what your sleep challenges are, know that you can overcome them. With dedication, patience, and determination you can finally achieve the restful sleep you need. You may stumble and fall along the way, but take heart in the fact that you now have the knowledge and tools to help you get back on track.

So take your newfound knowledge and use it to take control of your sleep. Don't be afraid to get creative, experiment, and persist. With a little effort and the right approach, you can finally conquer insomnia and find the sweet sleep you've been longing for.

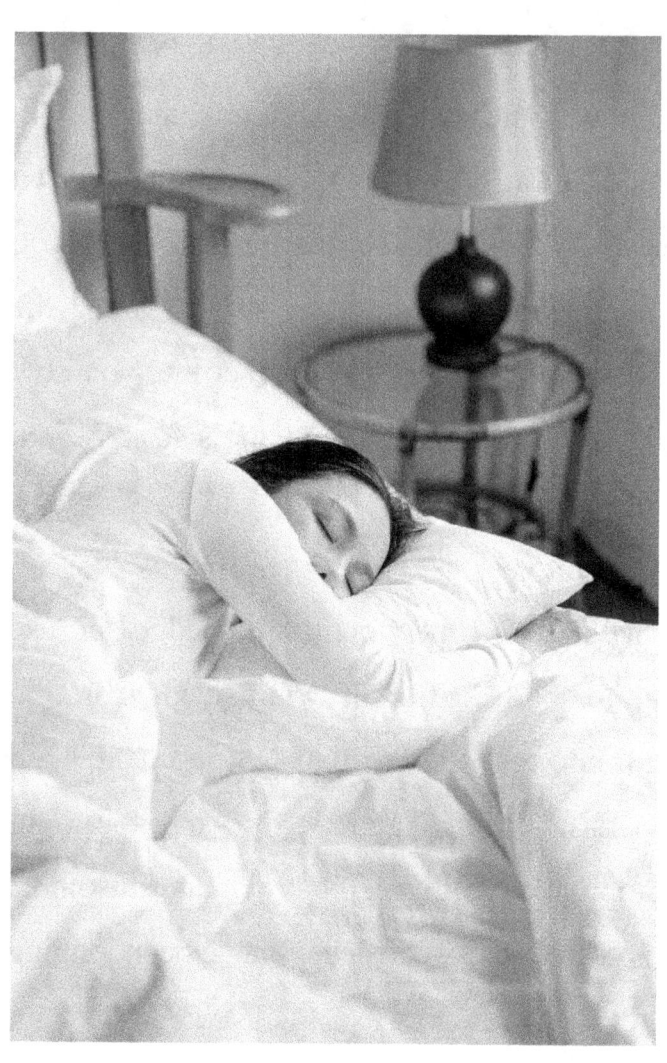